D1122658

THANK YOU, DR. LAMAZE

Thank You, Dr. Lamaze

by Marjorie Karmel

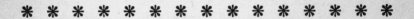

New Edition

HARPER COLOPHON BOOKS
Harper & Row, Publishers
New York, Cambridge, Philadelphia, San Francisco
London, Mexico City, São Paulo, Sydney

To the memory of Dr. Fernand Lamaze

All the names in this book are real, except for certain members of the medical and nursing professions in the United States.

A hardcover edition of this book is published by Harper & Row, Publishers, Inc.

THANK YOU, DR. LAMAZE *(New Edition).* Copyright © 1959 by Marjorie Karmel. Afterword copyright © 1981 by Harper & Row, Publishers, Inc. Foreword copyright © 1981 by Elisabeth Bing. "A Lamaze Manual for the '80s" by Marilyn Freedman, copyright © 1981 by Harper & Row, Publishers, Inc. All rights reserved. Printed in the United States of America. No part of this book may be used or reproduced in any manner whatsoever without written permission except in the case of brief quotations embodied in critical articles and reviews. For information address Harper & Row, Publishers, Inc., 10 East 53rd Street, New York, N.Y. 10022. Published simultaneously in Canada by Fitzhenry & Whiteside Limited, Toronto.

First HARPER COLOPHON edition published 1983.

ISBN: 0-06-090996-X (previously ISBN: 0-06-014831-4)

83 84 85 86 10 9 8 7 6 5 4 3 2 1

Contents

Foreword

"It is not only that I have been spared the pain and anxiety that my ignorance and fear might have caused me. It is more than that. I know that . . . I have got in touch with my essential humanity, that something truly beautiful has been added permanently to my life." These extraordinarily true words appeared in 1959 when *Thank You, Dr. Lamaze* was first published. Marjorie Karmel, the author of this beautiful and important book, felt more than twenty years ago that she had to find her inner self and find it through the most exciting and important events in her life: the births of her children, Pepi and Marianne (and, subsequently, Philippa).

How many of us these days talk about "finding ourselves," taking time off from studies to find out who we are, to make sure of our most precious heritage, our humanity. But how few of us think of finding ourselves while experiencing one of the most fundamental and peak experiences in a human life: giving birth.

When I came across Marjorie's book, I was at a time in my life when her philosophy touched a responsive chord in me and answered many doubts and questions. The publication of her book, and subsequently meeting and working with her, represented a milestone in my life, something I stumbled across almost by chance which fitted into my thinking at the time. Marjorie showed me that pregnancy and giving birth when shared through communication with one's partner can be one of the greatest of life's experiences for both mother and father.

More than twenty years have passed since Marjorie Karmel wrote this book, and its publication in 1959 was one of those extraordinary happenings in life that have repercussions impossible to foresee. American women and their partners were apparently so inspired by *Thank You, Dr. Lamaze* that they became the proselytizers of an entirely new approach to childbirth.

True, there was Grantly Dick Read with his philosophy of a painless childbirth through obliteration of fear, ignorance, and tension. But it took someone like Marjorie Karmel, with her determination, her perseverance, and her wonderful sense of humor, to inspire so many men and women to decide to change the whole approach to childbirth in the United States—to make it human, dignified, exciting, and gratifying.

I am sure that Marjorie could never have realized in her wildest dreams that her book would be the inspiration for millions of parents. Her spirituality and her love for humanity won the day and gave the whole obstetric profession a new direction.

Obviously, many changes have taken place since the author wrote this book. Changes in medical techniques, which have become extraordinarily sophisticated, ensure greater safety for both mother and infant than was possible twenty years ago. Relatively recently, too, research has shown that tobacco and alcohol present a risk for the unborn baby. Mention of Marjorie's occasional cigarette and martini remains in this new edition of her book—in fact, not a word of her original text has been altered—though I am sure she would have taken no such chances with her unborn babies' health if she had known what we know today. But in general, the amazing fact remains that Marjorie's ideas have not been superseded. They have been added to, they have been enlarged, and they have become guidelines for many childbirth educators, doctors, and nurses—guidelines leading in many different directions. Her ideas have become the overwhelming factor in keeping medical technology from swamping parents and making childbirth and parenting into an occurrence that has lost its soul.

Having taught the Read Method of Childbirth for several years, I wrote to Marjorie Karmel immediately when her book appeared. She telephoned me and said, "You must start teaching the Psychoprophylactic Method of Childbirth [Lamaze method] right away, because I have had hundreds of phone calls, letters, and even wires asking me to teach women to have their babies with joy and active participation. Both Alex and I," she added, "have been inundated with calls for help."

And that is how it started: We met, liked each other, and within months I was teaching the Psychoprophylactic Method of Childbirth at the Mt. Sinai Hospital in New York City under Dr. Alan Guttmacher. Within another few months, a few doctors, childbirth educators, nurses, and enthusiastic parents joined us, and what is now known as ASPO, the American Society for Psychoprophylaxis in Obstetrics, Inc., was born. In the same year, 1960, the International Childbirth Education Association was founded, as well as the La Leche League, both organizations whose aim it was to further family-centered maternity and good nursing conditions. Marjorie's ideas fell on fertile ground.

If Marjorie Karmel were with us today—she died far, far too early, in 1964—she would be in the forefront of all of us who are continuing to work for a humanized maternity, a family-directed maternity, an experience that we can remember in old age with the words, "I had a wonderful birth, and I got in touch with my humanity when I gave birth to my children."

Thank you, Marjorie Karmel.

Elisabeth Bing
Clinical Assistant Professor
Department of Obstetrics and Gynecology
New York Medical College

PARIS * * * * * * * * *

1 *In Spite of Myself*

"I'm not the type," I said when someone suggested I write a book about my experience with the Pavlov method. By this I meant that I am not the type of woman who feels compelled to spout out the details of her most intimate physical experiences to everyone who comes her way. I knew that the birth of each of my children had been a joyous and moving experience, and that this had been made possible by the way they were delivered; but after all they were *my* children—I couldn't expect anyone else to feel the same way. Still, after the idea had rattled around in my head for a few days, my conscience began to bother me. I felt that I owed a debt to the people who had taught me how to have children in this wonderful new way. But Dr. Lamaze is dead, Mme. Cohen is happily at work in her sunlit room high over a gray Parisian courtyard, and I don't even know the names of most of the others responsible for developing the method. The only way I can begin to repay my debt is by passing on to other women the experience that they made possible for me.

The Pavlov method is a technique of natural childbirth based on the conditioned-reflex theories of the famous Russian physiologist. Developed in Russian hospitals, it has become the preferred and nearly universal method of childbirth practiced in the Soviet Union and Communist China. It was introduced to France in 1951 by Dr. Fernand Lamaze, and immediately became a source of heated controversy for reasons having more to do with its country of origin than with its medical merits or demerits. Fortunately most of the wind was taken out of the sails of the political opponents of the method when on January 8, 1956, in a speech delivered at the Vatican before seven hundred gynecologists of fourteen nations, Pope Pius XII endorsed it as a "benefit for the mother in childbirth" which "fully conforms to the will of the Creator." But in the United States, so far as I can determine, it is unknown to all but the few obstetricians who pay attention to foreign developments, and it is practiced nowhere. Which is a damn shame, considering what a wonderful thing it is.

But then how much does anyone in this "enlightened" country of ours know about childbirth? When I look back at what I knew about the subject only a few years ago, I am appalled at my ignorance. I consider myself a fairly sophisticated person. My high school was noteworthy for its intellectual intensity and wild parties, and as for Bryn Mawr, my beloved second home, it is renowned for turning out super-educated women. Naturally I would have been surprised if anyone called me ignorant. Yet my ideas about childbirth were limited to some very vague notions about how hospitals and "advanced medical science" had solved or were just about to solve whatever the problems involved had been, and I considered the whole subject of no interest to anyone outside the medical profession. What I really meant, I suppose, was that it didn't interest *me*. When I look back now at that state of apparently carefree innocence, I see that it was only a very thin covering over a wealth of misconception and fears. And again I am reminded of my debt to the Pavlov method. It is not only that I am no longer ignorant, no longer afraid; it is not only that I have been spared the pain and anxiety that my ignorance and fear might have caused me. It is more than that. I know that with its help I have got in touch with my essential humanity, that something truly beautiful has been permanently added to my life.

I've always been skeptical about proselytizing. Not only is it often in poor taste, but it is usually ineffective. I don't think it is possible to sell something to anyone who doesn't already want to buy—probably because I have faith in my own powers of resistance. I consider myself impervious to the hard sell and the soft sell; if I don't want something I don't take it, not even if they're giving it away. I came across the Pavlov method by accident. I listened to the claims that were made for it and said, "Show me!" But then, to my surprise, I was shown—not only shown, but convinced and led into one of the greatest experiences of my life. This is the story of the rewards I reaped by letting myself be persuaded that I had something to learn.

It all began one cold night in England when we ran out of shillings to push into the heating machine in one of those overquaint English country inns. A few weeks later we were back in Paris, where we had been living for some time. Suddenly I began to feel nervous and upset. I gave up wine for a few days. In France wine can explain a lot of things. But I continued to feel peculiar. I even began to consider going around to a doctor. Then suddenly I was struck by an idea. I sat down with a calendar and did some rapid calculating. I waited a few more days and then decided that it must be true.

"Wonderful!" Alex said when I told him. "What do we do next?"

"I haven't any idea."

"I suppose you ought to see a doctor," he suggested vaguely.

"I suppose so," I answered. "An obstetrician. But where do we find one?"

We asked around and finally made an appointment to see a highly recommended obstetrician in the sixteenth *arrondissement*. As Alex drove me over, we suddenly realized that we were in for an experience that neither of us knew anything about.

The waiting room was an example of high-ceilinged French elegance. For some reason the other women seated about us all appeared to be approaching middle age. The atmosphere was hushed and solemn. The only sound was an occasional rustle as somebody turned a page of *Réalités*. After five minutes I began to feel uneasy. Finally it was my turn. We went together into a tremendous office fitted out with splendid furniture. The doctor, a thoughtful and soft-spoken gentleman, invited us to sit in two large leather chairs across the desk from him. When he had extracted enough material from us to begin a respectable dossier, he invited me into still another room to be examined. When that was done, he informed me that the delivery would take place at the American Hospital and that I had nothing to worry about. Until that moment it hadn't occurred to me that there might be anything to worry about. Suddenly his air of gravity convinced me that childbirth was a serious matter. I was relieved to find myself in such good hands. All I had to do was to start knitting little things and the rest was up to him. My only responsibility was to show up once a month for an examination. Wasn't Science wonderful!

A few days later we received a telegram about a serious illness in Alex's family. It was necessary for us to return to New York for some time. I called the doctor to cancel my next appointment.

"How do you plan to go?" he asked me.

"We're flying," I said.

"No," he answered. "You must go by ship. At this time it would be dangerous to fly. Aside from that you have nothing to worry about."

So Alex flew and I took the Queen Elizabeth home through one of the worst tempests in North Atlantic history. What with one thing and another five or six weeks slid past before I remembered that I was due for another examination. I called one of the best hospitals in New York and asked for the name of a good obstetrician. The woman at the other end of the line said she couldn't recommend doctors, but I finally persuaded her to read me a list of some of the men on the staff. As she read I jotted down five names that sounded euphonious. Then I put one hand over my eyes, made a mark on the paper with a pencil, and chose the name closest to the mark.

This time the office was on Park Avenue. It was essentially like the French doctor's office, only translated into American terms—read low ceilings for high, compact for spacious, modern for antique, and thirtyish women for fortyish. After a short wait, I was finally let into the doctor's private office, where I supplied the information for my dossier all over again. "I took a ship home," I explained when I got to the part about having returned to New York.

"Why didn't you fly?" the doctor asked me.

"The doctor in France said it wouldn't be wise," I said, much surprised.

"Some physicians are very old-fashioned, Mrs. Karmel," he answered with just a hint of condescension in his voice. "You will find that attitudes toward pregnancy have changed tremendously in the past ten or twenty years, and that a pregnant woman can do anything she would do if she were not pregnant. These days a woman can very nearly go through a pregnancy without being aware that she *is* pregnant." He chuckled benevolently, as if he had just told a backward child that there was no such thing as a goblin. "Do you drink?" he asked me.

"Yes. Some."

"I see that you smoke. Well, there is no reason to change your habits. Just enjoy yourself and leave the rest to me."

That was the sort of talk I liked to hear. I shook his hand happily and was about to leave. But I was a little bothered by what he had said about my French doctor. He had been very highly recommended, and I was planning to have the baby in France, not New York.

"Make Mrs. Karmel a reservation," the doctor said to his nurse as he showed me out.

"Oh yes, Mrs. Karmel," the nurse said. "Would you like private or semi-private?"

"But I told you I probably won't be here for the delivery," I said.

"You can always cancel," the nurse explained. "It's my opinion that you'll like a private better. There's very little difference in price and the rooms are lovely."

"Then I'll take a private," I said. As I wasn't going to use it, the price was irrelevant. I walked out into the street feeling very satisfied with myself. I had done more than my duty. I had two obstetricians and two hospital reservations. Aside from the little question as to which doctor was right about flying, I had nothing at all to worry about—even if I wanted to worry.

In this carefree spirit I went off to the fateful cocktail party which was to be the first step toward an unforeseen adventure. Almost as soon as I arrived, I was cornered by a young lady in an advanced stage of pregnancy. It was the third time I had seen her that way. Horrors! I thought. She knows I'm going to have a baby, and I'm going to have to listen to advice on child-rearing. (I had already promised myself that motherhood was not going to elimi-nate the rest of my life.) I was just preparing to ward off any talk of Spock or Gesell, when she caught me off-guard on the childbirth line. I was dumfounded. Childbirth belonged to the obstetrician, and I didn't see any reason to discuss it at a cocktail party. Obvi-ously American life had changed while I was away. I listened in as-tonishment while she went on and on about someone named Dr. Dick Grantly or Grantly Read—I couldn't make out which —and being fearless about childbirth.

"But really, I am fearless about it," I protested, as soon as she let me get a word in.

"That's what *you* think!" she said with the look of someone who knows better. "Besides, that's not the point. The point is the no-anesthesia part. You get to watch the baby be born."

"Watch what?" I asked. I felt sure I hadn't heard correctly.

"The *birth*," she repeated. "You get to watch it in the mirror."

"No, thank you," I said. "I'd rather not."

"But it's very beautiful," she answered. "You ought to try it. I can lend you the book."

The whole thing seemed improbable. "Did you really have your children that way—I mean . . . no anesthesia . . . and looking in the mirror . . . ?"

"Oh heavens no!" she answered. "My doctor doesn't believe in it. But I did read the book and it's so fascinating. It's so helpful. It really does eliminate fear. Do let me give it to you!"

I slipped off toward the canapés as soon as I could. My first exposure to natural childbirth had not been promising. I filed the subject in the remotest corner of my mind, with no intention of pursuing it further. If it really was a significant development I was sure my doctors would mention it when the time came. After all, they had been to medical school and I hadn't.

Several weeks later I was having lunch with the mother of a fourteen-year-old boy. By this time it was becoming difficult to hide my condition.

"I have a book you must read," she said almost as soon as we sat down.

"Really? What about?"

"It's about natural childbirth," she said. "*Childbirth Without Fear* by Grantly Dick Read—an Englishman."

"I think I've heard the name," I said. "What's so appealing about his book?"

"Appealing? It's just thrilling! I'm going to send you my copy. I know you'll like it. You'll probably want to try it yourself by the time you get to the end."

"What makes you think that?" I asked. "Did you?"

"No," she said, "I hadn't heard about it when John was born. But seriously, please read it. It's just inspiring!"

I was beginning to wonder what there was about me that invited these attacks. Why should people feel compelled to interest me in something they hadn't even done themselves? I felt I was being pressured and I didn't like it. I was not interested in natural childbirth—not even if they were giving it away.

"I don't like inspirational literature," I said.

A week later the book arrived in the mail. It sat on the desk and gathered dust for several weeks.

We made our plans to return to France. We decided to go by ship because we liked it better, and bought our tickets. The night before we left, we packed our suitcases. "What about this?" Alex asked, holding up Dr. Read.

"What about it?"

"Do you want to take it?"

"I'll never read it."

"Are you sure? Nine days is a long time."

"Well . . . throw it in then."

In went Dr. Read, between *The Brothers Karamazov* and the brothers Grimm. Down went the lid. In the morning we set out for the dock in a spirit of lighthearted anticipation. We were about to have nine peaceful, sunny days at sea. We had no idea of the emotional dynamite we had so casually flung into our suitcase. No one had suggested to us that Dr. Read was capable of causing a storm at sea.

2 Doctors Read and Lamaze

For the first three days the weather was lovely. It wasn't until the middle of dinner on the fourth day out that I was seized by the compelling necessity to go below. I dived into bed fully clothed and reached out for something to distract my mind from the disturbing activities that were taking place in my stomach. The dull tan cover of *Childbirth Without Fear* was not particularly inviting, but at the moment it didn't make much difference to me what I read. The ship heaved and trembled; one book was as good as another. I opened to somewhere in the middle and glanced at the top of the page. . . .

"Let us consider what happens to a girl in a maternity home for her first baby . . ." It was an intriguing consideration. I had never consciously thought about the question before. "She probably has every care and attention from the purely obstetric point of view, but is it often remembered that nothing is more terrifying to her during her first labor than being left alone . . . ?" Another interesting question. "Two, three, or even four women lie together, some quietly bearing the unexplained sensations; some suffering pain; some crying out in sheer terror with each contraction. . . . At length, with her spirit almost broken by the assault of agonizing doubts and fears, she is deemed ready for the final stages. . . . She then finds herself being led into such a room as she has never seen before. In spite of her condition, she notices in the twinkling of an eye her surroundings; the nurses, and perhaps the doctor, draped in long white gowns, white caps and masks. . . . She does not fail to notice the glass-fronted cupboard in which hangs a large collection of instruments; she has heard of instruments, but had no idea that they looked like that. . . . Then she climbs upon a high bed, harder and more uncomfortable than any she has ever known. . . . She lies in whatever position she is told. I wonder if the average man can even imagine the thoughts that would go through his mind if he were subjected to a similar experience?"

Never, I thought, never in this world! In one page I had been won to the cause of misunderstood womanhood. I was in a fever of anxiety; the *mal de mer* had vanished. Something more acute had come to take its place.

Alex came down much later. "I thought you were going to sleep," he said.

"What? Oh . . . later."

He climbed into the upper and switched off his light. I read on. When I got to the end of the book, I immediately turned back to the beginning. I was in the middle of the preface when Alex switched on his light again.

"Go to sleep," he said, "or you'll feel worse tomorrow."

"As soon as I finish," I said.

"Finish it in the morning." His light went off again.

I decided he might be right. I turned off my light and tried to sleep. Inside me the baby began to kick and jiggle. I was wide awake. The book was tucked into the corner of the bed sending out electric signals. I listened to the sound of the waves sloshing against the side of the boat. I was acutely awake. I turned on the light again and returned to the book.

By the time I had finished, I was extraordinarily excited. Dr. Read's book, in spite of its title, had left me the victim of a tumultuous host of fears. But I couldn't blame them on Dr. Read; his book had not created them. Rather I felt them called up from some place deep down inside myself where I had been hiding them. I had repressed every fearful thought, realistic and imaginary alike, because I wanted to be strong. Now they all came flooding up together, and I was going to have to look at them. Nothing in the book seemed improbable to me when I remembered my past experiences with hospitals and doctors. My head was crowded with ideas and impressions. I was quite thoroughly terrified—but at the same time I felt curiously relieved. I was glad to have come face to face with my fears now, rather than have them suddenly confront me when I was in labor. And the fact that there was someone like Dr. Read in the world who knew about such fears and sympathized with them, was, in itself, tremendously reassuring.

I lay awake trying to think what I was going to do. I couldn't imagine myself having natural childbirth because I felt I was too cowardly to risk feeling any pain. I believed Dr. Read when he said that pain did not necessarily accompany childbirth, but I was sure that I would become tense and create it for myself. I had such a long history of sitting rigid and anguished in the dentist's chair that I couldn't imagine myself smiling peacefully through the long ordeal of labor. On the other hand, I desperately wanted to remain conscious for as long as possible and most of all I wanted not to be left alone. "Don't exaggerate," I told myself, "you're not the first person who ever had a baby." But then all sorts of fragments of stories I had heard and presumably forgotten came rushing back into my head, and I knew that I could not possibly rationalize away my fears.

A gray light began to filter in through the porthole. The cabin gradually grew lighter and lighter. I heard sounds of stirring above.

"Alex?" I asked softly, more to see if he was awake than to awaken him.

"What's the matter?" came the answer from above.

"Would you mind very much being there when I have the baby?"

"Are you still reading that book?"

"No, I finished it long ago. Did I ever tell you what happened to my mother?"

"No."

"She was left alone after the delivery. My father happened to walk in and notice a pool of blood under the bed . . . it was dripping right through the mattress. Mother wasn't even breathing—they had to revive her with the rescue squad. What would have happened if he hadn't been there?"

"You never told me that before."

"I hadn't thought of it before. Of course, it was only an accident, but I wish you'd stick around anyway."

"Don't worry," he said, "we'll arrange it with the doctor as soon as we get to Paris."

"What if he won't let you be there?"

"Then we'll find another doctor. That seems to be a pretty upsetting book you're reading."

"It is upsetting," I said, "but it's great. Why don't you take a look at it?"

I handed up the book and heard him begin to turn the pages. My insomnia went with it. I didn't wake up again till lunchtime. Alex was just finishing the last chapter.

We discussed the book at great length all afternoon. The one thing we found we could not share was Dr. Read's profoundly mystical view of the spirituality of motherhood. I wanted to have my baby very much but I did not feel I could get rhapsodic about giving birth. I doubted that I could waft myself through the experience without the assistance of an anesthetist. But I was thankful for the knowledge that would enable me to approach the experience in a rational manner instead of being subject to all the fears that I had found hidden away in myself.

That evening we won at horse-racing and then danced late into the night. When I finally got to bed, I was tired and happy, and quickly fell asleep. A few hours later I found myself awake and in the middle of a mental dialogue on the subject of anesthesia.

"Alex?"

"What?"

"Do you think anesthesia really works?"

"Of course it works."

"I had a wisdom tooth pulled with Sodium Pentothol, and when I woke up I was crying. I had a cut sewn up with gas, and I can still remember the hideous nightmares I had. I had a broken back set under something else, and I remember being terribly upset afterwards. The intern said I made a frightful racket. It must have hurt me dreadfully."

"What difference does it make? You didn't know about it if it did."

"Some part of me knew. I'm convinced that some part of me suffered excruciatingly. . . . And also, I was wondering . . . have you ever thought about their mixing up the babies . . . ? I mean, that you might accidentally get the wrong baby at the hospital."

"As a matter of fact I have. But you don't have to worry, I'm going to be there."

"You know, I think I'd like to try it. What can I lose? They can always give me something if I make a mess of it, but I want to see that baby right away and know it's mine. I don't want to be somewhere else having a nightmare when he's born. . . ."

"Listen," Alex said, "we'll stop in on the Clays while we're in Holland and ask them about their doctor. Then if we can't find anyone who does this thing in France, we can have the baby in The Hague."

"Why the Clays?" I asked.

"Don't you remember? They had their first baby in Rome and it was gruesome. The second one came when they were at The Hague, and Jack insisted on being with her. The doctor was wonderful, and all she had were a couple of whiffs of gas."

"Really? I didn't know that!"

"You do so know it! You're amazing. You seem to have managed to repress the whole subject!"

I was astonished. We had spent a whole evening listening to the Clays talk about their experiences with childbearing, and I had totally forgotten every word of it until that minute.

Our first stop in Holland was The Hague. The Clays were delighted to tell us their story again. This time I listened carefully to all the details. Jack assured Alex that it was a marvelous experience to watch the birth of one's own child, and not the least bit upsetting. I privately asked Mary if she wasn't at all embarrassed about having Jack watch—as much as I wanted Alex to be there, the idea seemed just a little unromantic—and she assured me that she was not. They promised to arrange things for us in The Hague if we found it impossible to work something out in Paris. After that we plunged into a week of sight-seeing, confident that things would work out well.

Mary Clay had not taken any preparatory training course, but she had been allowed to have Jack with her in the delivery room, and *he* had been allowed to give her the few whiffs of gas she needed whenever she had asked him for it. She had been fully conscious for all but a few seconds during the delivery. This was not like the method Dr. Read outlined in his book. Nor was it exactly like many of the methods I later came across that professed to be based on Dr. Read's work. The Pavlov method, which I eventually found in Paris, was less like Dr. Read's doctrine than any of the others. In the United States most of what is called natural childbirth is more or less based on the work of Dr. Read, usually with many important modifications. I have a tremendous respect for Dr. Read and his accomplishments—I suppose that is obvious from the strength of my reaction to his book. But the fact remains that I couldn't go along with his rhapsodic and mystical view of childbirth, and, as Dr. Read explains, it is precisely this mystical view that is responsible for the truly successful deliveries performed according to his method.* The Pavlov method, as I will describe further on, replaces this emotional force with a whole series of physical and mental techniques based on the conditioned-reflex and pain theories of the Russian physiologist I. A. Pavlov. The differences between the Read and Pavlov methods are not merely theoretical; they are practical as well. They exist in almost

---

* "We see the rejuvenating pregnancy of women who have faith in the mysterious force that guides them safely through the intricacies of the great adventure." *Childbirth Without Fear* p. 97. "When exhilaration and intense joy are experienced physical changes occur which are readily diagnosable at sight and strangely infectious. The ecstasy of love that floods the whole personality when the earliest call of new life awakens a woman to the realization of motherhood, is a transport akin to mysticism." *Ibid.* p. 98. "Elation, relaxation, amnesia and exultation are the four pillars of parturition upon which the conduct of labor depends." *Ibid.* p. 142.

every phase of the training the expectant mother receives as she prepares to embark on the adventure of having her baby. The modifications of the Read method which are performed in the United States are even further removed in theory and practice from the Pavlov method (but I will save that for Part II). What is common to all systems of natural childbirth is the belief that much of the pain and distress that so often accompany labor is caused by fear, fear created by widespread misconceptions and by the thoughtless and inhumane organization of many lying-in hospitals. All these systems attempt to eliminate fear by educating women and by reorganizing the institutional setup. Of course I didn't know anything about all this even after our evening with the Clays. All I knew was that Dr. Read's book had convinced me that it was possible for many women to have babies without anesthesia and without much pain, and although I did not have much confidence in my ability to go through with it, I was by now determined to try to have mine that way.

After a week of looking at more Rembrandts and Van Goghs than we had ever thought existed, we got on the *Nord Express* to Paris. As soon as we were comfortably resettled on the Place Maubert, we went to see our general practitioner. When he heard what we wanted, he laughed heartily.

"Now you don't *really* want to go in for all that stuff, do you?" he asked, wrinkling up his nose with amused distaste.

"Oh yes, I *really* do," I persisted.

"I suppose someone here does it," he admitted frankly, "but I certainly wouldn't like it for *my* wife." He raised an eyebrow and turned to Alex. "And I couldn't bear to be around to watch either!"

He suggested that before we do anything else we visit the American Hospital in Neuilly and a maternity hospital called the Château de Belvédère, decide which décor we preferred, and reserve a room. In the meantime, he promised to look for a doctor indulgent enough to go along with our bizarre desires. He laughed

good-humouredly as we said good-bye. It was obvious that we af-
forded him no end of amusement.

We went to the Belvédère first. It really was a former château
of Louis-Napoleon vintage. It was just across the Paris city line
near the Porte Saint-Cloud and was surrounded by a charming
garden where we caught a glimpse of a few terribly pregnant
women and their husbands walking up and down and enjoying
the sun. It seemed very remote from the bustle of Parisian life.
The directress, a decisively authoritative woman who looked like
the headmistress of a fashionable girls' school, showed us about.
Each room was more delightful than the last. All of them looked
out on the garden, some had balconies, some fireplaces, and in
each one was a cradle hung with white ruffles and topped with a
pink or blue bow. Looking at all that charming provincial décor,
it was difficult to remember that we were really in a hospital. I
was just beginning to wonder if we hadn't wandered into a country hotel by mistake, when the directress pointed to a heavy metal
door bearing a sign that ordered us in no uncertain terms to stay
out. Beyond that door, she informed us, was the modern delivery
wing. Just then a young nurse came to call her to the telephone.
The directress marched away, leaving us in the care of the new-
comer, who was much less prepossessing. I immediately used the
opportunity to ask her if she knew anything about natural childbirth—had it ever been done in the clinic?

She looked at me with such astonishment that I was sure I had
committed some dreadful indiscretion. Then suddenly she broke
out into a torrent of enthusiasm that severely taxed my French.
The main gist of it seemed to be that she had seen it practiced,
that it was very often practiced right there in that very clinic, that
she had seen it with her own eyes, that it was the latest thing, that
it was very daring, very efficient, *très splendide, émouvante, profonde, et très, très belle!*

Well then, I suggested, perhaps she would be able to tell me
the name of a doctor who practiced it.

"Alas no," she sighed, unfortunately it was not her province to recommend any particular accoucheur. She was desolated.

"Alas," I sighed back, however was I going to be able to enjoy that *émouvante* experience?

Suddenly she brightened. She could, she remembered, give me a list of all the accoucheurs who regularly used the clinic.

I had just remarked that perhaps it might be possible for her to underline one or two of the names on the list, when the directress rejoined us. I quickly changed the subject. I felt as though I had just escaped being caught smoking in the dormitory.

We went to the office to discuss the fees. We were given some literature and a long list of things I was to bring to the hospital when the time came. Finally we were turned back to the custody of the nurse to be shown to the door. As we started down the steps she stealthily slipped a little folded paper into my hand. "*Bon chance!*" she whispered, and closed the door behind us. We waited till we were in the car to look at the paper. On it we found two names—Dr. Pierre Vellay and Dr. Fernand Lamaze.

"How do we choose?" I asked Alex.

"Flip."

We decided to look at the American Hospital before we did anything decisive. We drove up to Neuilly and looked around. The American Hospital was big, impressive, and American. The rooms were equipped with hospital beds, sparklingly clean and white, earnestly austere. The whole place very clearly said NO NONSENSE. We were back in the lobby trying to decide whether or not this more businesslike atmosphere implied medical superiority, when whom should we see but our own doctor. We waved to him.

"What are you doing here?" he said, when we got his attention.

We reminded him, and he laughed again. "Come along to my office and have a chat." He led us down a side corridor. "I did ask around," he said, "and as preposterous as *I* think it is, I've nonetheless found the man you are looking for. The name is . . .

now what the devil is his name? Well, I wrote it down somewhere . . . where . . . hmmm . . ."

We waited patiently while he ruffled papers, looked under
paperweights, lit a cigarette, and scratched his head. It was an
elaborate production. "It's Lamere, or something like that. . . ."

"It isn't Lamaze?" I asked.

"Exactly! Lamaze! Fernand. He's famous for that sort of
thing—he invented it, or if he didn't invent it—anyway he does
it."

"Seriously," I said, "do you recommend him as an obstetrician?"

"I wouldn't tell you his name if I didn't," he answered,
smiling blandly.

Looking back now I see that it was not such an extraordinary
coincidence that he and the nurse at the Belvédère had hit upon
the same man, but in the brightness of that Paris afternoon it
seemed as though Fate had pointed the way. We went immediately to the nearest telephone, looked up Dr. Lamaze in the
Bottin, and called for an appointment.

Two days later we walked down the boulevard Saint-Germain
to the rue du Dragon. We were in the heart of Saint-Germain-
des-Près, halfway across Paris from the fashionable Passy apartment house where our first obstetrician's office had been. We
found number 21, and went through a dark passageway that
led to a shady little courtyard. The entrance to Dr. Lamaze's
office was not prepossessing. I looked at Alex doubtfully. "Let's
have a look anyway," he said, and I rang the bell. We were
ushered into a dark, cluttered room that did not look as though it
was intended to be a waiting room. When my eyes adjusted to the
gloom, I found we were in the company of several other women
and a few husbands, all of whom were sitting stiffly on uncomfortable, old-fashioned chairs. The room was full of books,
Buddhas, paintings, and an assortment of unidentifiable bibe-
lots. The total effect was curious and rather musty. We waited
nervously, wondering whether we hadn't stumbled onto some

charlatan. What doctor had a waiting room like this? After about an hour, we were told that the doctor would see us.

There in another room very like the first, only smaller and darker, stood a rosy-faced, blue-eyed man, who seemed to me like a magical creature in a children's book, ready to lead us on to a new adventure. "I am Dr. Lamaze," he said in French. "What can I do for you?"

The answer seemed obvious to me, but I began anyway. "I have read Dr. Read's book . . ."

"That is different," he cut me off. "Dr. Read's method is *accouchement sans crainte*—childbirth without fear; I give you *accouchement sans douleur*—childbirth without pain. Are you interested?"

I was a little confused. "I don't understand," I said.

"During my visit to the Soviet Union in 1951 . . ." he began.

We listened with growing astonishment as he gave us a short account of how he had first heard of the Pavlov method of painless childbirth during an international conference on obstetrics in Paris in June 1951 and how later the same year he had observed it being practiced in Russian hospitals. He had been so impressed and thrilled by the deliveries he had witnessed there, that on his return to France he had immediately begun to practice the method. The Read method, he explained, is based on the theory of eliminating tensions caused by fear, and thereby letting nature take its course unhampered by harmful emotions. The Pavlov method, while it agrees with the principle of conquering fear by knowledge, also makes use of conscious mental and physical control of the birth process. This control is attained through exercises and education designed to build conditioned reflexes which will stand up during the stress of labor and enable the woman consciously to direct her own delivery. "You have your baby yourself," he concluded. "I am only there to assist you." From my limited experience with doctors this struck me as unparalleled modesty.

That was the first I had ever heard of the Pavlov method. I knew the Russians claimed to have invented everything, but childbirth seemed an outlandish addition to the list. I was a little suspicious of the whole thing. I looked at Alex. He was wearing a slightly strained expression that suggested to me that he felt the same way.

"Will you step into this room, madame, and place yourself upon the table?" Dr. Lamaze asked politely. I went behind the hanging curtain at one end of the room and into the tiny alcove that he used for examinations. There was a sink and an examining table, but the shelves along the wall held more of the same collection of books and *objets d'art* that filled the rest of the office. I found this amusing, but at the same time it made me uneasy. I had never before met a doctor who was a humanist as well. Can this scholar really deliver a child, I wondered, or am I really going to be expected to do it all myself?

The examination was like the others I had had, except that all through it Dr. Lamaze kept muttering, "Good, good, very good." "Madame," he pronounced when he had finished, *"vous êtes parfaite!"* I wasn't sure just what aspect of me he was referring to, but it made me feel very good. "Monsieur," I heard him say to Alex as he went back to the office, "I find that madame is perfect." When I rejoined them they were deep in a discussion of French literature.

As he showed us to the door, Dr. Lamaze handed me a piece of paper on which he had scribbled a name and address. "This will direct you to Mme. Cohen," he said. "She will instruct you in the method. She speaks English. She will be your *monitrice,* which is to say that it will be she who will teach you the principles of our system and the exercises that will enable you to carry them out. You are just beginning the seventh month, you have plenty of time. Mme. Cohen will also be with you at the time of your delivery, and she and I together will assist you while you do the work of bringing your child into the world. We will act together as a team. It is a very beautiful thing to bring a child into the world, *n'est-ce pas, madame? C'est belle. C'est la plus belle chose du monde!*"

He looked at me expectantly. I thought of all the other beautiful things in the world. I tried to imagine what it must look like when a baby entered the world. I wasn't at all sure that *belle* was the best word for it. For a moment I felt I was being given a sales talk and I didn't like it.

"*C'est belle, madame, n'est-ce pas?*" he repeated.

I gave in. What difference did it make? "*Oui,*" I murmured, "*c'est belle.*"

"*C'est une expérience profonde,*" he went on, radiant with enthusiasm. "And as for your baby, he will be superb. He will suffer none of the harmful effects of drugs. You will know that you have given him the best possible start in the world. But now—" he cut himself short (clearly his enthusiasm tempted him to go on much longer)—"I will expect to see you again in a month."

We walked out into the sunlight fascinated but skeptical.

"Why not string along for a week or two?" Alex said as we sat down at a café. "Let's find out what it's all about. I don't suppose that politics can affect childbirth one way or another."

"I wouldn't miss it for anything in the world," I agreed. "And I liked what he said about the baby."

"Their system certainly has a confident-sounding name," Alex said. "I wonder if they aren't being a little overoptimistic."

"Childbirth without pain?" I answered. "Wouldn't it be delightful if it turned out to be true. . . ."

3 Do It Yourself . . .

The next morning I got up early and went out to the *tabac* to call Mme. Cohen. I bought a *jeton* and a pack of Gauloises and sat smoking and drinking coffee while I gradually worked up the courage for the phone call. Although I can understand almost anything in French, I don't speak it like a native and somehow when I find myself face to face with a telephone my vocabulary shrinks. I carefully constructed several elegant opening sentences. Then I got worried about subjunctives and discarded them all. Finally I picked up my *jeton* and the paper with the number on it, and marched into the phone booth prepared to take the plunge. I dialed the number and tried to think of what to say while it rang.

"*Allo,*" came a voice from the other end.

"*Je voudrais parler à Mme. Cohen, s'il vous plait.*" It really wasn't so hard as all that.

"And what can I do to serve you?"

"Dr. Lamaze told me to call you to ask—"

"Yes. Good. I understand."

"Dr. Lamaze told me that you understand French . . . oh, no, what I mean is . . . he told me that you can speak English. . . ."

"Oh! But no!"

It was a bad beginning. For a moment I was sorry I had not gone right to the American Hospital where everyone spoke English. While I had this unhappy thought, Mme. Cohen went right on talking. Then she stopped and there was a long silence.

"You are still there, madame?"

"*Oui, madame,*" I answered sadly.

"Tell me please, madame, you are English, isn't that so?"

"No, madame, American."

"All the same. Don't bother yourself about it. But listen carefully, madame. We will do very well together. You understand? I promise you. You may be sure of it!" She sounded so confident and cheerful that I supposed she must be right. Why shouldn't I be able to have a baby in French? I wasn't planning to have it by telephone.

"Now listen carefully, madame," she went on, "I am going to speak very slowly."

"Thank you," I said relieved.

"I will make you an appointment," she said, rounding out each word with fine precision. "Will you come to me here at eleven o'clock this Friday? Good. What is your metro? St. Michel? Excellent. Get on at St. Michel, go to Barbès . . . Barbès. Do you have a pencil? Good. Get out and cross the boulevard, turn right, you will find the house. You have my address? Good. Go through the doorway and cross the first courtyard. Enter the next doorway. On your right you will discover staircase A. Go straight up to the sixth. Now. Listen carefully. You must go up slowly. Each time when you arrive at a landing, stop. Rest for several seconds. Breathe deeply. Then continue slowly. Don't forget. Breathe deeply on each landing. Walk up slowly. Good. Is that perfectly clear?"

"Perfectly," I repeated. The little map I had drawn according to her directions had an improbable appearance, but I had followed every word she said, and no doubt it would get me there.

"Good. And you will bring your husband with you, no? Excellent. And one thing more, madame . . ."

I had broken my pencil point, and I wasn't sure I could remember one thing more.

"What is your name?"

"Oh," I laughed. "Madame Karmel. K-A-R-M-E-L."

"Very good. Madame Karmel. And madame, you have understood everything? Good. Then, till Friday!"

The instructions were absolutely accurate. We crossed through the little gray court, entered the dark passageway, and turned right into staircase A. As we cautiously began to negotiate the stairs, I was struck by the thought of Kafka as a realist. When we reached the sixth I was almost surprised to find that there actually was a door on which were cards confirming the existence of a Blanche Cohen, physiotherapist, and an Henri Cohen, photographer. We rang the bell. Mme. Cohen showed us into the living room to wait until she finished her previous appointment.

The walls were covered with beautiful photographs, obviously the work of Henri Cohen. The bookshelves spilled out periodicals. The apartment faced a courtyard on either side, but somehow the atmosphere was cheerful and, mysteriously, sunny as well. There appeared to be only two rooms and a kitchen, and I had the impression that Mme. Cohen, her husband and their child all lived and worked there.

We were shortly shown into what I can only describe as a sort of parlor-office-classroom. The center of the room was taken up by a high hard table such as one finds in a doctor's office or a reducing parlor. There was a daybed against one wall, and all around the others were cabinets, shelves and chests, holding stacks of paper and photographs and books. The walls were covered with photographs, and on a blackboard beside the high table was a diagram that appeared to be a fever chart.

Mme. Cohen was a young woman of medium build, slight, with short dark hair, and large dark eyes that rapidly switched their expression from a serious shyness to a delightfully mischievous sparkle. I liked her immediately. It was impossible not to. She spoke to us simply and earnestly, but from time to time she smiled in a way that made us feel we were sharing in some incomparably gay adventure.

At the sight of the high table in the center of the room, I immediately anticipated that I would be asked to climb up and perform some sort of ridiculous athletic contortion. I wouldn't have minded that terribly if it hadn't been for the presence of my husband. I was greatly relieved when Mme. Cohen asked us both to sit down on the daybed and proceeded to talk to Alex.

"I am happy that you could come today, monsieur," she said. "Although it is possible to succeed without you husbands, we much prefer to have your help. There is an important part for you to play in your wife's *accouchement*. I hope you will have the time for it, and I can assure you that you will come to feel that it has been time well spent. It is a great pity that a man should stand back, helpless and inadequate, *de trop*, while his wife alone knows the profound experience of the birth of the child they have created together. Even the man who is willing to come and watch his child be born, but will not share the work of preparation, is likely to feel as much an outsider to her experience as if he had not come at all. That is why I asked you both to come. Madame will come to me six times, at two-week intervals. If you come with her for the first three lessons, that will be enough. But you must help her practice at home, every day if that is possible —a half hour will be enough—and I hope you will be able to come with her to see our movie."

Then she turned to me. "For you there will also be a visit to the hospital where you will become familiar with the delivery room and have an opportunity to question one or two mothers who have already had their babies without pain. You must remember when you go to tell me your impressions of the hospital and the film. We are always looking for suggestions for improvement. Now, madame, let me find out something about you."

I was about to launch into that now-boring history that had already filled so many dossiers, when she explained that my medical records were the concern of Dr. Lamaze. What she was interested in was my knowledge and impressions of the facts of childbirth. As my knowledge was limited to some vague memories of diagrams I had seen in a biology class and what I had managed to get from Dr. Read's book, my impressions had so little to base themselves on that they didn't amount to much more than a sort of diffused anxiety. She seemed so pleased by my lack of information, that I must have looked surprised, for she immediately exclaimed "You see, we will not have to waste our time undoing misconceptions. Frequently, the women that I see have listened to so much advice from so many friends that we must *de*condition as much as we condition."

She took up a portfolio of plates and diagrams. We were to begin by a "review," as she flatteringly put it, of everything that happened from the moment of conception to the moment when the child was put into his mother's arms. Then we would consider how best we could effect and aid the process. I was a little bored as she flipped through the diagrams showing the embryo working its way down the fallopian tube to nest and grow in the uterus. I was overcome by the same sleepy feeling that had been responsible for my 68 in biology. Then as the foetus reached term and the time for the delivery approached, she shifted to a set of plates that quickly revived my interest. They were photographs of plaster models that showed the successive cross sections of the woman's body as the baby moved from the womb out into the world during labor. The first one showed the relative positions of the baby, membranes, and uterus at the onset of labor. The plates that followed showed how the uterine muscles pulled at the neck of the uterus (or cervix) and, helped by the pressure of the baby's head, first flattened it so that it seemed to disappear altogether, merging into the general shape of the rest of the uterus, then stretched it open little by little like the neck of a sweater until finally it was a circle wide enough for the head to pass through. The baby appeared to turn as it entered the birth canal.

To illustrate this Mme. Cohen took up a little doll and a model of a pelvis to demonstrate how the baby rotated to allow first the head and then the shoulders to pass comfortably through the bony structure of the pelvic cavity. I was aghast with admiration for the clever intricacies of nature. It had never occurred to me that birth involved such elaborate maneuvers. *"C'est belle, n'est-ce pas?"* Mme. Cohen asked us.

"C'est extraordinaire!" I answered.

"Now that we have this child in the birth canal, let's deliver him and put him away for a while. Will you make a circle with your hands? There. The head has crowned—become visible. This is how the doctor will deliver the baby." And she slowly worked out the doll's head, turning it up so that little by little the face appeared, first eyes, then nose, then all of it. She turned the child in place and extracted an arm, then another turn, and there was the second arm. Then she lifted the doll triumphantly through the circle of my hands, and put him to rest on the table.

"Are you sure it's that easy?" I asked skeptically. Clearly she must have oversimplified for the purpose of instruction. Her response was more than I had bargained for. She took a stack of photographs from the bookshelf and spread them out on the table. We had to stand up to look at them. At the first glance, my mouth dropped open and I nearly sat down again. She had set out in order a series of photos that showed minute by minute the emergence of the baby from its mother. The pictures were clearly of a real delivery; a real live woman giving birth to a real live baby. I had never even imagined what such a sight might look like, and I was so shocked and embarrassed that I could scarcely focus enough to see what she was pointing out to us. I glanced at Alex nervously to see what his reaction was. I could feel myself blushing. Strangely enough, Alex didn't appear to be the least bit disturbed by it. He gazed intently at the pictures, and seemed to be listening carefully to whatever Mme. Cohen was saying.

Suddenly she swept the entire series to one side of the table and replaced it with another. "There you are again," she said. "The head has crowned. Here you see the entire face, now the shoulder and arm. You see how the doctor has turned him. . . ." At last I had the courage to look. There it was, happening just as she had said it would, only it seemed impossible. I looked at the size of the baby's head, and knew that I could never go through with it. She had just talked me out of natural childbirth.

"The expressions are marvelous," I heard Alex say.

What could he be thinking of? I looked at the pictures again, and for the first time I noticed the expression on the woman's face. She looked excited, even rapturous, and there was nothing about her that suggested that she was feeling any pain. In the last picture she reached out for her child looking as though she might burst for joy. All the same, I couldn't really make myself believe that the expression on her face had anything to do with the rest of the picture.

"C'est belle, n'est-ce pas?" Mme. Cohen smiled.

Alex nodded. I began to think they were both crazy. I had a second of relief when she swept this set away, but when she replaced it with another, and still another, I could feel my irritation growing. The faces of the woman kept smiling, the babies kept coming out, Mme. Cohen kept talking, and Alex kept agreeing with everything she said. Every so often she punctuated her discourse with "C'est belle, n'est-ce pas?" and that enraged me. I did not think it was beautiful, far from it, and I was not going to be pushed into agreeing with her for anything in the world.

Suddenly I heard her ask if Alex had a camera. He said he did. "Very good," she exclaimed happily, "then if monsieur would like to—"

I saw what was coming. "No," I stopped her, "it isn't a question of what monsieur would like. Madame will absolutely not allow it."

She smiled sympathetically. "Certainly not, if you feel that way, but in later years you may come to regret not having a tangible record of one of the most meaningful experiences of your life." It was the same speech they had used to sell us wedding photographs. It was a logical extension of a common enough practice, but I couldn't conceive of doing such a thing.

"It really doesn't make any difference," she said with a smile, seeing that I had not taken kindly to her suggestion. "The important thing is having the baby. And now, I hope, you have some idea of just what we are referring to when we use the word *accouchement?*" I nodded quickly for fear that she would bring out more photographs if I said no. The first shock over—how little I really knew about my own feelings!—I was beginning to feel a certain amount of curiosity, but I did think that I had had enough for one lesson.

"Very well, then I shall go on to tell you something of just what your role will be in this matter. Because even though childbirth is a perfectly natural process, it is not something that you simply let happen to you. That is not sufficient. Rather it is something you *do.* And to do it well, you will have to learn to control your body so that it can work efficiently and painlessly for you, and you will have to learn to control your mind so that it will remain in good working order throughout the whole process. My job is to help you learn this. But first I am going to tell you something about the scientific base on which our method rests. You have heard of Pavlov and conditioned reflexes? And perhaps of Pavlov's famous dog who was trained to salivate when a bell rings, no?"

Again I was reminded of the biology course I had nearly failed. I vaguely remembered something about a dog, but not just what it was supposed to prove. I looked at Alex who was nodding as if he understood every word. I figured he would explain it to me later.

For readers whose recollection of the famous Pavlov experiment may be as vague as mine was, here is a greatly simplified explanation.

It is noted that a dog salivates at the sight of food. This is called a fundamental reflex. For a number of times a bell is rung whenever food is put in front of the dog. Then it is noted that the bell alone without the food produces salivation. The fundamental salivary reflex has been conditioned to respond to a new signal, the bell. It is now a conditioned reflex.

"Very well," Mme. Cohen went on. "That of course is an example of a fundamental, built-in reflex that has been *conditioned* to respond to a new signal. It is also possible to condition reflexes so that the original signal provokes a new response. Much of what we shall be doing in these lessons will be building up conditioned reflexes that will be useful during your *accouchement*. For example, I am going to teach you a way to push by blocking air in your lungs and bearing down with your diaphragm that is far more effective than the way you would instinctively push if you were left to yourself. When, during your delivery, nature sends you the signal to push, you will automatically push the way you have been taught without having to think about it. But we shall make use of more of Pavlov's theories than just that. Again and again I will remind you of Pavlov's insistence that the whole of your nervous system is a physiologic unity, that all your sensations—including pain—and all the things your body does—including the functioning of your internal organs—are controlled by that part of the brain we call the *cerebral cortex*, that is by the surface of the topmost part of the brain. You will be training muscles, yes, but that will be the smallest part of your work. Most of the time you will be working on your brain, developing its inherent capability to control your body and suppress pain—in a word, *conditioning* it to enable you to do what you have to do to have a truly painless childbirth. That is why we do not call our system 'natural' childbirth. The final result should be better than nature. And now, shall we get to work?"

After all that, I was afraid I was going to be called on to do something tremendously difficult. Fortunately we began with some simple exercises designed to develop general suppleness and muscular tone. I stripped to the slip and climbed up on the exercise table. The idea was simply to lie flat on the back alternately raising the legs as high into the air as possible, taking the longest possible time about it, and then lowering them with record slowness. A dance class I'd had in college now paid dividends. I didn't even have to be told to keep my knees straight. Mme. Cohen smiled approvingly.

"As you find that so easy," she said, "let us proceed to the next one. Please extend your arms to the sides at right angles to your body—like this—now lift your right leg and swing it out to the side in the direction of your right hand. Very good. Excellent! *Formidable!* You American girls are extraordinary, aren't you? So supple, so athletic. This exercise is usually accompanied by moans and lamentations. French girls can be such a lazy lot. You will do these a few times every day, and when you have the opportunity, sit like a tailor. You know how? Very good. These exercises are to help you now; they aren't for use in labor, although they will prepare your body to function at its best when you most need it. They serve to limber the joints that must stretch in the delivery, to increase the elasticity of the pelvic floor, and to keep your circulation from being sluggish. They are also helpful in preventing muscle cramps and varicosities. Have you ever had a muscle cramp? No? Then we will hope you will not have one now, especially during your delivery. They can be very threatening to your control And now let us move on to some exercises in muscular control."

"But is that the whole calisthenic?" I asked, surprised.

"Yes," she said, "you need not be an acrobat to have a child."

I waited confidently for her instructions. By now I was certain that I would excel in muscular control.

"This exercise, you will see, is training more for the mind than for the body. Tense your left leg and right arm simultaneously. The right leg and left arm must be completely relaxed."

I smiled and nodded before I had really considered what she had said. Then I repeated it to myself. "Aha! Yes, I get it." It took me nearly a minute to get each of my extremities into the required state.

"Very good," she said, testing my tense arm and leg, "but why do you find it necessary to make that ferocious face?"

"I'm concentrating."

"Try to concentrate while smiling like Buddha," she suggested. "Now let's see how the relaxed extremities are doing." She tested them. They weren't relaxed. She shook them slightly until they were limp enough to meet with her approval. By that time the supposedly tense arm and leg had slumped into a similar state of lethargy. Eventually I achieved the proper arrangement of alternate but simultaneous tension and relaxation. "Excellent," Mme. Cohen pronounced. "Now when I give you the order to reverse, you will immediately relax the left leg and right arm and tense the others—with no faces, please. You must learn to reverse the entire process without having consciously to think about it, automatically and all at once. Now, reverse." My performance was chiefly distinguished for its confusion. Alex laughed. (When he tried it himself later, he apologized.)

"Is that supposed to be an exercise in relaxation?" I asked. "Because, if it is, it had just the opposite effect on me."

"We do not want to achieve 'relaxation' in the American sense of the word," she answered. "You must not think of it as taking it easy. That would be too passive. That would only slow down the activity of your brain, which in turn, as I will explain later, would increase your sensitivity to pain. Instead of 'relaxing,' you must learn to let go of your muscles consciously and actively, so that *they* are at rest, but your mind is not."

That made sense to me. It sounded like what my modern-dance teacher meant when she taught us to contract and release. When I relaxed I was usually on the edge of sleep. To release, on the other hand, was to be very wide awake.

"That is why I did not speak of relaxation exercises, but of exercises in muscular control," Mme. Cohen continued. "You are going to learn to direct your muscles to respond to a given signal. It will require an active mental effort on your part. Again now, left leg and right arm tense. Everything else relaxed."

I snapped back into the first position.

"Reverse," she said. It took me nearly a minute to get reassembled. "Don't look so discouraged," she said. "How many years did it take you to learn to read and write? You didn't consider yourself hopeless because you had to go to school? You didn't despair because you were born ignorant of the multiplication table? Of course not. Certainly not. And yet you expect to control your body perfectly the first time you ask it to perform in an entirely new way? No. You can't create a conditioned reflex without constant repetition. One concentrated effort is not enough. You must train yourself to make your body respond in a specific way when you give it orders. This is how you will *learn* to have a child. It is a learning process. You will learn to give birth the way you learned to read. When the time comes you won't have to think about how to do it. You will be fully rehearsed, and your mind will be free to concentrate on your performance."

"Now," she continued, "I would like to try to give you some idea of how a labor contraction will feel to you, and how you will control it. You know that the contractions pull the cervix open and force the baby's head against it at the same time. When that is accomplished they push the baby out into the world and the placenta after him. You have seen the mechanics of the thing. But what will your sensations be while this long process is going on? What will you feel? What will you do? Remember that in the first and longest part of the labor, the uterus will be engaged in pulling open the cervix until it is a circle wide enough to permit the passage of the baby's head. Each of the contractions that does this will be a strong muscular sensation that will begin slowly, giving you sufficient warning of its presence, then mount more or less rapidly to a maximum peak, after which it will decline sharply. Here is a picture of an average contraction."

She snatched up a piece of chalk and outlined another dramatic-looking fever chart on the blackboard. The tiny ups and downs in the graph she explained as representing the pulsating quality of an extreme muscular tension.

"What will your feelings be as this occurs?" she continued. "Imagine that you are at the seashore. You see a great wave begin to gather up far out from the shore. It is obviously going to pass over you. There is no escape. As it approaches it grows higher and higher, gathering force. If you turn and run, you will be knocked down and pounded by the surf. You will certainly be hurt. If you remain facing it, eyes shut, in an attitude of fear and helpless surrender, you will most certainly become rigid as a stick of wood when the wave strikes; you will be swept under, pulled about in the undertow and, ultimately, even drowned. What should you do? You must observe its course calmly, with your eyes fixed on it every second. As it approaches you, you swim above it, for your calm has given you the energy and mental alertness necessary to time your strokes and use your strength to its greatest advantage. As you feel it pass beneath you, you smile and sink slowly to the ground, with the knowledge that you will be able to repeat your performance again and again, as long as the waves continue to come. You will experience the pleasant thrill of victory. But if you panic—you will be submerged. This chart is the outline of that wave. Today I will teach you how to master the rather gentle waves of the sort that are considered the pleasantest for surf-bathing. Actually they occupy a large part of the first stage of labor."

At this point she tucked a pillow under my head and produced a long round bolster, or *traversin*, from somewhere in the corner

which she placed under my knees. I felt so relaxed and comfortable that I was in danger of falling off to sleep. I automatically
sighed and shut my eyes.

"None of that," she said. "I can see you have never been to
the seashore. No experienced vacationer ever takes a nap in the
surf. Now, during this period the uterus does not require any
active assistance on your part, in fact it would very much prefer to
have you stay out of the way as much as possible. In this respect
it will demand your utmost cooperation. It is not an easy thing to
provide your uterus with this maximum noninterference. You must
maintain a state of relaxation in which your mind is alert and in
control of the rest of your body. And you must breathe in a way
that will keep you on top of our metaphoric wave. Now take a
deep breath."

I was just about to give another demonstration of the excellence
of my artistic education, when she stopped me short.

"Not like that!" she said. "Why are you pushing your stomach
out that way?"

I made a brief speech on the virtues of abdominal breathing
to which she listened very patiently. "Perhaps for singing," she
commented. "But remember that here we have set ourselves the
goal of not disturbing the uterus while it is at work. What will
happen if you come pushing down on it with all that air?"

"Then how am I going to take a deep breath?" I asked in-
dignantly. I had spent so many years perfecting my abdominal
breathing. I didn't want all my work to have been in vain.

"The rib cage is capable of great expansion," Mme. Cohen
explained. "Here, and here, at the sides, and here at the top. If
you lift your chest—shoulders at rest please—you will find that
you have room for a large quantity of air. Like this."

She inhaled slowly through her nose, keeping her lips closed
tight. It was astonishing to watch the expansion of her chest; everything below her waist remained perfectly still. Then she slowly
blew the air out soundlessly through her mouth, much as if she

were blowing up a very fragile balloon. The air entered and left her chest in a slow steady stream. It was tremendously yogi. My imitation, on the other hand, was tremendously Sad Sack. My shoulders moved up, my diaphragm down; I made an inelegant hissing sound, and I finished the circuit in about half the prescribed time. Nevertheless she smiled at me pleasantly and assured me it would come. Then she took up her stop watch.

"We will assume that your contractions are coming every four minutes for a duration of fifty seconds. I will tell you when you first see the wave. You will breathe in this manner, evenly and rhythmically until it has passed under you and subsided. Ready. Begin. Five . . . ten . . . twenty . . ."

By the count of fifty I felt pleasantly dizzy. "Rest," she said, "breathe normally. Four minutes have passed. Begin." After a few more contractions, she told me the work was finished for the day. I started to rise. "No," she said, "don't get up immediately. You are not accustomed to so much oxygen. When you practice you must be sure to rest before you stand up. Otherwise you may find that you feel faint."

"Is that all, really?" I asked, surprised.

"For today," she said. "Do all Americans always want to learn everything at once?" We laughed.

I looked at my watch and saw to my surprise that we had been there over an hour and a half. It seemed as if we had just come. Mme. Cohen made an appointment to see us again in two weeks, and we trooped down the six flights feeling excited and trying to remember everything she had said.

For two weeks we practiced regularly and enjoyed the Paris springtime. In a few days I had mastered the exercises and they took very little of my time. Alex helped me by calling out "reverse!" and testing to see if my arms and legs were truly limp or tense as they were supposed to be. He timed my breathing for me too, and eventually evolved a system whereby he could read, looking up every now and then to call a command or test a leg. We had got the idea of collecting a complete set of an old edition of the *Comédie Humaine* which gave us an excuse for long walks on the *quais*. I also took advantage of my status as a pregnant woman to make Alex drive to the Halles to buy me oysters and *oursins* at improbable hours of the night, although this often resulted in his making long detours via Saint-Germain-des-Prés that brought him home hours after I had gone to sleep. All this was pleasant enough, but underneath I felt a growing impatience to go back for my second lesson. More than that, Mme. Cohen's description of childbirth had been a challenge to my sporting nature. I was beginning to feel eager for the *accouchement* itself.

4 . . . *In Six Easy Lessons*

When we arrived for the second lesson, we forgot all about breathing deeply on each landing and raced straight up the six flights without stopping. As we collapsed breathless and puffing onto the daybed, Mme. Cohen took up a piece of chalk and began to scribble something on the blackboard. I watched her fascinated— more fever charts. "Here," she said handing me a pencil and some old photographic paper, "I want you to copy what I write. If you lose it, don't worry. I'll write it out for you many more times. Writing is an excellent way to learn." It turned out to be perfectly true. She was going to write out the same thing many times, and

with diagrams. The last copy I received from her crossed the
Alantic in the mail a few weeks before my second child was due.
It is now permanently fixed in my mind.

"The whole process of childbirth, as you know, falls into two
main parts—the flattening and dilatation (or opening) of the
cervix, and the expulsion of the child and the placenta. The moment when the dilatation ends and the expulsion begins is a very
complicated one, and is often called the phase of transition. We
will talk about what you do during the expulsion later. What I'd
like to give you now is a diagrammatic summary of the contractions you will have up to and during the phase of transition and
of the techniques you will have at your disposal to use at each
stage."

With that she turned to the blackboard and pointed to the
first fever chart, which looked like this:

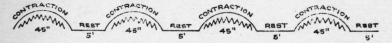

"This is a representation of the contractions that dilate the
cervix until the opening is about the size of a five franc piece
[fifty-cent piece]. These contractions may take several hours to do
their work, and when they begin they may be so mild that you
may not feel the need to do anything about them at all. When
they become stronger, you deal with them by doing the slow and
deep breathing that you have already learned. You may add to
this a slight *effleurage*—light massage—of the abdominal region.
I will show you how to do that in a little while. You notice from
the diagram that these contractions take forty-five seconds and
that you have five minutes to rest in between."

She looked over my shoulder to make sure that I had taken
down what she said correctly, then turned back to the blackboard and pointed to the second chart:

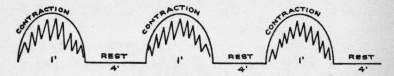

"These are the contractions that take the dilatation to about the size of the heel of your hand. You notice these are stronger than the others and mount in a crescendo like a musical phrase. They last one minute, and you have four minutes to rest in between. At some point during this phase the slow and deep breathing will prove inadequate to keep you swimming confidently on top of the wave. Then you will switch to an accelerated breathing or panting, which we will practice later on today, and go on with the *effleurage*."

The next diagram looked like this:

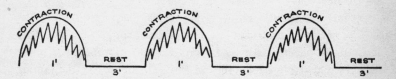

"These," Mme. Cohen said, "are the contractions that take you to a dilatation the size of the palm of your hand. You notice that they are stronger than the others, and that you have only three minutes in between. You go on with the accelerated breathing and the *effleurage*, and make very sure to take full advantage of the time you have for rest."

The last diagram was more complicated than the others:

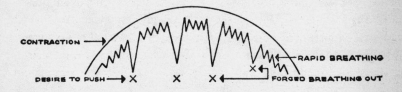

"This," Mme. Cohen said, "is a representation of a single contraction during the phase of transition. The phase of transition
lasts from the time the dilatation is at a full palm until it is large
enough to permit the passage of the baby's head. It is complicated by the fact that your nervous system, anticipating a little, is
already sending you signals that give you a strong desire to push.
These signals are represented by the sharp dips in the graph that
I have marked with an X. But if you obey these signals and push
now, the result will be painful because the cervix is not yet open
wide enough to let the head pass. So what you do is continue the
accelerated breathing and punctuate it with a strong blowing out
whenever you feel the desire to push. In this way you will be able
painlessly to get through what is often a difficult moment. Now,
is all this clear to you?"

"It seems a little too clear," I objected. "Or do you mean it to
be a general abstraction of what might take place? I don't suppose that anything always works that regularly."

"Oh no," she protested, "you will be surprised to find how
accurate everything actually is. The amount of time each phase
requires is variable depending on the individual. But the timing
of the contractions is normally a constant. Chance really has very
little to do with it; it is all ordered like a ballet."

Having seen a few off nights at the ballet, this last statement
left me not entirely convinced. But I was in a hurry to get on to
the exercises.

Alex looked on proudly while I astonished Mme. Cohen with
the results of our practice. To my delight I found that I had
completely mastered the muscular control. Seeing that the original
exercise was now so easy for me, Mme. Cohen added three more of
the same type in rapid succession. My body responded amazingly;
I was surprised to find that even on a first try it was no longer
difficult to do what was expected of me. When she said right arm
tense, it immediately was so. My brain had learned to respond
to that particular set of commands in a broader context than I

had imagined. Mme. Cohen looked delighted. "You are going to be a great success!" she exclaimed.

Then she pointed to the first diagram on the blackboard. "The contraction is about to begin," she announced. She clocked me while I did my slow breathing. "Excellent," she pronounced. "Now we will add the *effleurage*. Let me demonstrate, first on myself and then on you."

The *effleurage* turned out to be a very light massage of the area just above the pubic bone, the place where the contractions were likely to be felt most intensely. It is hardly accurate to use the word massage to describe it. It was a light stroking, in a circular pattern, that felt as though a butterfly had condescended to brush his wings across my skin. Mme. Cohen arranged my hands in a position where they were held up, not resting on my body, just over the pubic bone, the fingers touching the skin ever so lightly. First, though, she sprinkled the area with talc to avoid irritation of the skin. Then she guided my fingers lightly out toward the hip bones on either side, up over the area of the contracted uterus, then down to meet again at the starting place. The sensation sent a shiver of delightful relaxation out over my entire body.

"At home you will practice this alone and with the breathing," she explained. "In labor it will be performed from the beginning of each contraction, starting simultaneously with the breathing. It is very important to coordinate them both in perfect rhythm. Let me see you try. Go!"

I coordinated them all right, but the timing of the breathing ceased to resemble anything that could be called a rhythm. It was like being asked to sing the Star-Spangled Banner while rubbing your stomach and patting your head at the same time. "What good is all this in labor?" I asked plaintively.

"You will see," Mme. Cohen explained. "We are attacking on several fronts at once. The *effleurage* will relax the abdominal muscles in the region of the cervix which tend automatically to become tense during a contraction. The breathing will increase the supply of oxygen without interfering with the action of the uterus, and keep your blood richly oxygenated. We suspect that much of the pain of labor is caused by the fact that the extraordinary activity of the uterus exhausts the supply of oxygen in the blood. There may be a chemical reaction resulting from this, an accumulation of toxic substances, that causes pain and might be responsible for a sort of cramp that many women experience as an unending state of contraction. This has not yet been firmly proved, but all of our experience points that way."

"It's worth a gamble then," I said. "But why do you keep talking about rhythm? What difference does the timing make so long as I get the oxygen?"

The rhythm turned out to be the most important point of all. As no one had yet managed to understand all the possible causes of pain in labor, a certain amount might persist despite all the mechanical precautions of relaxation and oxygenation. This residue of pain had to be combatted at the place where it was perceived—namely, the brain itself. "The brain," Mme. Cohen explained, "can never be aware of *all* the sensations that are constantly being sent to it. If it were, it would be incapable of doing anything other than merely perceive. This means that whenever the brain is engaged in an activity, it shuts out many of the sensations that are sent to it. This shutting out or inhibition of sensations is referred to as *raising the sill of sensibility*. The greater the activity of the brain, the higher the sill of sensibility will be, the stronger a sensation must be before it can distract the brain from what it is doing. Thus," she went on, "a man who is running a race, his mind entirely fixed on the goal of winning, may fall and bruise himself severely without being aware of any pain—he will get up and go on running as if nothing had happened. It is only afterwards, when the race has been run, and his mind is no longer concentrating so intently on what he is doing, that he will become aware of just how much his scraped leg hurts. The rhythmic breathing and the activity of relaxation serve the same purpose during a contraction as the goal of winning the race. With your mind concentrated on them—on swimming above the wave—your sill of sensibility will be raised, and any painful sensation arising in your uterus will be inhibited. This is why, in the exercises I gave you to do last time, I stressed that what was desired was conscious control, not generalized relaxation."

We reviewed the exercise a few times. Then Mme. Cohen held up her hand for me to stop. "Listen!" she said. I could hear the loud hammering of a workman somewhere in the court below. "That's very well timed!" she exclaimed.

"Why?" I asked. It seemed anything but that—hammering always annoys me.

"Did you hear that noise when you were doing the exercise? No? And yet it was going on all the while." She looked at Alex and he nodded. So what? I thought. "The center of excitation that you created in your cortex by performing the exercise acted to inhibit your reception of that other excitation. Now that you have stopped, the other excitation can claim its share of attention. You see, this is one of your most effective weapons against pain, and it is entirely in your control."

I was astonished. So that was why I had to begin at the very beginning of each contraction, and that was how I was to stay on top of it. For the first time I had a real sense that I was going to have an active hand in making my labor painless. Suddenly I felt the baby inside me begin to kick and jiggle. "He's terribly active today," I remarked.

"Why not?" Mme. Cohen smiled. "He feels good. All that oxygen makes him want to play."

She pointed to the second diagram on the blackboard. "Now," she said, "the contractions are getting results. They begin to get stronger and stronger. The sensations they create are increased in intensity and threaten to overwhelm you and turn into pain. Now you must reinforce your defenses. Watch! Here comes a contraction!"

She drew in a long deep breath, then blew out every cubic millimeter of it. Then she began a rapid, superficial breathing, light, soundless, apparently involving little more than her breast-bone. She continued soundlessly for sixty seconds by her watch, then exhaled in relief and smiled.

"Contraction over," she said. "I have lifted the mechanical activity of breathing even farther from the uterus, because now the uterus would be truly resentful of any interference from the diaphragm. I have quickened my breathing to compensate for the loss of oxygen, and I have increased the concentration and rhythm so as to strengthen the center of excitation in the cortex. You try it."

It looked easy. I inhaled, exhaled, and began to pant. Within ten seconds my rhythm faltered and I began to feel strangled with breath. My shoulders and abdomen shook violently with every puff. I quit in despair. The second time I began, Mme. Cohen put her hand on my chest and told me to think of pushing it rapidly up and down. She did the exercise herself to accompany me. I managed to get through thirty seconds. Sixty was out of the question.

"Don't try to put this together with the *effleurage* until you have mastered the sixty seconds," she warned, "you won't be able to do it. This is your most important weapon, and you must practice it as often as you can."

"The baby keeps kicking me," I interrupted. She put her hand on my abdomen. "No," she said. "You're having a contraction. Here. Put your hands here and feel it."

"Does that mean I'm having premature labor?" I asked, shocked.

"No, no. The uterus does this very often. It's warming up. It's a muscle after all; it likes to exercise as well as you."

The contraction gradually faded away. I tried to remember if I had ever felt such a thing before; if I had, I must have thought it was the baby stirring.

"But if that's all a contraction is," I exclaimed, "I don't understand what all the fuss is about. That was nothing."

"That contraction, remember, is not a labor contraction. It is serving quite a different function. In labor, the contraction will be doing its job on the cervix. It will follow this mounting curve to a much greater intensity." She pointed to the blackboard. "But you will find this contraction very useful nonetheless," she went on. "You can study it so that you become expert at catching it at its very beginning. Whenever you feel one coming, practice your breathing with it. That way, when you are in labor you will already be trained to begin your activity early enough always to be ahead. The excitation from the uterus will never get over your sill of perception, and you will never lose control."

She looked at her watch, and we realized that once again we were overtime.

Practicing the accelerated breathing was much more difficult for me than the muscular control exercise had been. Nevertheless, by the time two weeks had passed I had mastered it. Alex had become accustomed to having a huffing grampus for a wife. By now the idea that there was any other way to have a baby had vanished from our minds.

The third class began with a review. Mme. Cohen corrected whatever she found wrong with my performance before going on to new material. Then she asked me to do the *effleurage* at the same time as the rapid breathing and, much to my surprise, it was an easy thing to do. From then on I was always to practice them together. If I found myself short of breath, I was quickly to exhale all the air I could and begin again. I tried this once or twice. When I had mastered it, she went to her blackboard, erased the diagrams that were left there from her last pupil, and again drew the fourth of the diagrams she had made me copy the time before.

"This, as you remember, is a contraction during the phase of transition," she said. "The cervix is almost completely dilated, but not quite. Nature, in anticipation of the next phase, has already begun to send out signals for you to begin to push. This is the most difficult moment in labor. These signals are the first step in what we call an absolute reflex, that is, one you have *not* learned, but that is already built into your nervous system. For that reason it will be very difficult not to respond to these signals. But if you push too soon, it will be painful. What we are going to do now is build up a conditioned reflex that will combat this ill-timed desire. When you feel this sensation, you must let the doctor know, and go on with your light, rapid breathing. Whenever you feel the urge to push, you must exhale forcefully. That will make it impossible for you to push. You must be more alert than ever, your control must be complete. You must go on doing this until Dr. Lamaze or I see that the head has passed through the cervix, and give you the command to push. Let's try it. When you feel the urge to push, you will say '*Ça vient!*'—Here it comes! The answer will probably be '*Pas encore!*'—Not yet!"

It turned out to be an easy exercise to practice. The urge to push was purely imaginary.

"Next," Mme. Cohen went on, when I had performed that to her satisfaction, "we are going to turn to the most active phase of the delivery—the period of expulsion. The work you will do now will be the most demanding and the most rewarding as well."

She took away the pillows that I had practiced with so far. The object of this was to reproduce as nearly as possible the conditions of the delivery itself. That is why the lessons were all conducted with me on a high table and Mme. Cohen standing over me. We would be in exactly the same relationship at the time of the delivery. Similarly, when the expulsion period began, the pillows would be taken away from me.

She helped me get in position with my knees bent, legs drawn up and spread apart, feet flat on the table. (In the delivery room there would be stirrups instead.) When I felt the contraction or a desire to push, I was to announce *"Ça vient!"* or "Here it comes!" Then if Dr. Lamaze gave me the signal to push, I was to take hold of the bars (in practice my own legs) and, lifting my head and shoulders slightly from the table, I was to pull against them. At the same time, I was to take a deep breath, blow it out, take another, hold it, and push down on my uterus with all the force of the air in my lungs behind the push. Thus the muscle of the diaphragm would add its force to the muscles of the uterus in expelling the baby. When I felt a need for more air, I was to exhale quickly, inhale again, hold, and continue to push. With practice I should be able to learn to push for seventy seconds without taking a breath more than once or twice. I was strictly warned not to exert my full force in practice. Instead I was to puff up my belly so as to get the idea of the action without really exerting much pressure on the uterus.

"Whenever you're ready, madame," Mme. Cohen said when she had completed her instructions. I felt a little foolish. I looked at Alex, and he nodded expectantly. Here goes, I thought to myself. *"Ça vient,"* I said aloud.

"Pas encore, madame!"

I hadn't expected that, but I remembered in time and began to pant, blowing out every so often to indicate that I really would like to begin to push. Mme. Cohen smiled happily, and again I announced *"Ça vient!"*

"Allez-y, madame. Inhale . . . exhale . . . *Inspirez . . . soufflez . . . inspirez . . . bloquez . . . poussez . . .* POUSSEZ POUSSEZ POUSSEZ POUSSEZ POUSSEZ POUSSEZ . . . *soufflez . . . inspirez . . . bloquez . . . poussez . . .* POUSSEZ POUSSEZ POUSSEZ POUSSEZ . . . CONTINUEZ . . . CONTINUEZ . . . *et soufflez. Reposez-vous. Très bien, madame. Très bien!* You will be a formidable pusher. FOR-MI-DABLE!"

Mme. Cohen rustled about some piles of paper and finally came up with a little pad and pencil which she handed to Alex. She made him write down the little pushing dialogue word for word to use in our home rehearsals. "Keep it," she said, as he was about to hand back the pencil. "We haven't yet come to the end of the scene."

"Now," she said, turning back to me, "let us analyze the way we have been pushing. It is a way we have arrived at experimentally and which we find very efficient. When we first began we found that when we told women to push, they pushed the way they do when they make a bowel movement. Now, how is that?"

I looked at her blankly. "Think about it," she persisted. "Now do it and tell me what you feel."

"Well . . . I sort of tighten my stomach, I guess, and hold my breath . . ."

"Exactly," she said. "You pull in your abdomen and tighten the muscles of the perineum. If you did this at the moment of the expulsion, it would have the effect of pushing down on the uterus and compressing it laterally, and at the same time, closing the door through which the baby is to make his entrance into the world. It is inefficient, and can be painful as well. That is why I want to warn you about that bad association with pushing. When you practice the exercise I have just taught you, you must always be sure that the perineum is relaxed. You must do all your pushing with the diaphragm, with the whole force of all the air blocked in your lungs behind it. You must repeat this exercise correctly until it becomes a reflex. A fast expulsion is the best thing for your baby."

"Does the way the woman pushes really make a significant difference in the time?" Alex asked.

"She can cut the time in half," Mme. Cohen said. "In terms of the health of the baby, this is probably the greatest advantage of our method."

She reached into a drawer and pulled out a stack of pictures.

They were the same ones that had upset me so during our first visit. This time I was able to look at them more calmly.

"Now we will examine the second moment when nature sends you a command that you must not obey." She pointed to the first picture. "Here the baby's head has just crowned. At this moment I will say '*Ne poussez plus*'—Stop pushing. Will you write that down, monsieur? At this moment, madame, you must lie back and do the rapid, superficial breathing. That will prevent you from pushing."

She glanced at Alex's paper to make sure he had written her command correctly. "Why do we ask you not to push at this moment? Here is the head. It is pressing against an opening which is not yet large enough to let it pass. If you push now, the force of your diaphragm behind the baby may make the head tear the delicate tissues of the perineum. You must lie back, panting and relaxed, so the doctor will be able to perform his delicate task of working the head slowly out without any pain to you."

She put down the picture and picked up the doll she had "delivered" during the first lesson. She outlined a circle on its head. "This is the way the head presents itself when it first crowns. Notice that it is the largest diameter of the skull which is turned to the opening. Instead of letting the head be forced through directly, the doctor will gently work it back and lower it so that the first part to emerge will be a smaller circumference at the back."

She lowered the doll's head to illustrate the angle at which the head would be delivered. Then she turned to the next picture which let us see the moment in real life. There was no longer any question of being shocked.

"Now," she went on, turning from one picture to another, "the doctor slowly lifts the head up and out. Here you see the eyes, now the nose, now the entire head is clear. Monsieur will be able to look into his baby's face, even before madame."

"No!" I interrupted, my last bit of feminine modesty coming

to the surface, "monsieur will stay up at the head of the bed. He can see the baby's face when I do."

Mme. Cohen misunderstood my reason; she thought I was jealous of Alex's seeing the baby first. "Never mind," she said consolingly. "Dr. Lamaze will keep you informed of every step as it progresses. He will announce to you 'forehead, eyes, nose,' etc. You will know just what is going on. Now, here he is turning the baby, and here he is delivering the arm. 'Madame,' he will announce to you, 'here is your baby's arm.' You will feel it on your thigh. You may lift up your head and look into your baby's eyes now, even before he is completely born. Here."

I looked at the photograph before me. For the first time I really understood the expression of joy on the woman's face. She could feel the little arm against her leg, and she was getting her first glimpse of the face of her child.

"After that the rest of your child will slip out easily. You will be able to see whether it is a boy or a girl. A moment later you will hold him in your arms, and on that happy note, let us finish for today."

The fourth lesson was a total review of everything I had learned so far. We took each exercise separately, and discussed when it was to be used and for what purpose. The basic education had been completed. What was left to do was to enforce the new reflexes I had acquired.

The fifth took the form of a rehearsal. We moved straight through an imaginary labor, at each step reviewing the probable time involved, the sensations I might have, and the techniques I would be able to employ. When I finally arrived at the end of the expulsion and was holding the imaginary child in my arms, Mme. Cohen explained how the doctor would cut the cord and how a few moments later I would expel the placenta with a push or two. "That's all there is to it," she said. "A normal birth is an uncomplicated affair."

"It's just delightful," I agreed. "Nothing to it!"

"I said uncomplicated," she corrected me. "Not easy. Don't forget for a minute that it's going to be very hard work. If you do, you're going to be badly surprised. Remember it's called *travail*. What is the word for it in English?"

"Labor," I answered.

"And what does that mean?" she asked.

"Hard work," I said.

"You see it is the same. Don't forget it. It is the hardest work you will ever do in your life. But unlike so much work, this work will be rewarding."

She went off to look for the paper on which she had written the dates of the movie I was to see and the hospital visit, and I sat back and marveled at how much I had learned. "Be sure to take monsieur to the movie," she reminded me when she came back. "And now, before you go there are one or two things I want to tell you about the hospital. When you go there you will see a large tank at the head of the table in the delivery room. It is nothing poisonous—only oxygen. It is there in case you fall behind in your breathing or for some reason do not get enough oxygen. I will give it to you by holding a mask over your face between contractions. You'll notice the mask is made of plexiglass. We used to have a rubber mask, but some women said they felt psychologically stifled by it. The plexiglass is transparent."

She reached into a drawer and pulled out a funny-looking instrument, rather like a pair of calipers. "If the membranes have not ruptured by themselves by the time you are at five francs dilatation," she explained, "the doctor may use this instrument to rupture them for you. You won't even feel it. But there is one important thing to remember about the rupturing, whether it occurs naturally or artificially—immediately afterwards the contractions will become much stronger and closer together. You will have to be especially alert; the rhythm of the contractions may suddenly change. Try to analyze the new rhythm as quickly as you can. I'll be there to help you if you threaten to lose control. Now, enjoy the movie, and I'll see you again in two weeks for the dress rehearsal."

All through the ninth month, I was getting larger and larger. Spring had turned into summer. Alex and I had spent an afternoon getting acquainted with French baby clothes and buying a supply. We even bought a delightful musical doll we saw in a store window one afternoon. My due date was only a week away, but even that now seemed like a long time to wait.

"Have you packed your suitcase?" Mme. Cohen asked me as I walked in for my final lesson.

"Should I have?" I asked, wondering if there was something about me that made her think I was going to give birth then and there.

"Pack it tonight," she said smiling. "Be sure to include some talc for the *effleurage* and a sponge to wipe your face if you get hot. Another thing. When your due date comes around, I want you to shave yourself. Don't look so startled. Use a mirror and do it yourself. Otherwise they will have to do it for you when you get to the hospital. If you are having strong contractions, it will interfere with your control. When you are just about to set out for the hospital, give yourself an enema. That way they won't have to give you one at the hospital when you are further along in labor and might find it both unpleasant and disturbing."

Really, she thought of everything. I wondered if the Russians were so considerate. She went on to enumerate the signs of the beginning of labor and the procedure I would follow checking into the hospital. When I got there, I was to be sure to ask any questions that occurred to me, not to puzzle over anything that I didn't understand. If I were not very far along, I might knit, walk in the garden, sleep, or talk, whatever I found most restful. But I was not to do anything that would tire me for the work that was to come. I understood that Alex could be with me the entire time, and that there would be midwives and nurses in and out periodically to check on my condition. Mme. Cohen herself would arrive when I was approaching five francs dilatation, and Dr. Lamaze shortly afterwards, before I had reached transition.

"Before our final rehearsal," Mme. Cohen went on, "there are several things I want you to keep in mind. One: Go on practicing every day. If you are overdue, you will come for another lesson. You have built up temporary conditioned reflexes. You must stay conditioned and not let them fade away. Two: Rest and save your energy as much as possible. Don't turn up exhausted. Fatigue lowers the sill of perception. Remember, when you are tired you say 'Everything gets on my nerves.' Please do not come to your *accouchement* in a state of exhaustion. Three: Remember that you are entering a competition that you are going to win. The first stage, the dilatation, may be long, hard work, but you will be alert and in control. When you reach the expulsion and feel the baby slowly move down with each of your pushes, you will know that the victory has been well worth all the time we have spent together. We are working as a team—you, me, your husband, Dr. Lamaze, and the staff of the hospital. Each of us has a part to play. Yours is the most important of all. Now, let us rehearse."

We went through the whole thing twice. The second time we threw in an extra push for twins—just in case. I had gone through it all so many times, at home with Alex calling the signals, and here with Mme. Cohen, that I was confident that when I was finally in labor, it would work nearly automatically. Then suddenly, from somewhere in my subconscious, despite all those weeks of training, out popped an old nagging question.

"Will there be anesthesia just in case?"

"The hospital will have anything you want," Mme. Cohen laughed. "But do you really think you are going to need it?"

"No," I said, "in fact I know I won't—now that I know it's there."

We discussed an American movie she had recently seen and the Moiseyev ballet, both playing in Paris at the time. (Mme. Cohen liked the movie and labeled the ballet *tarte à la crème*.) Then we said "Au *revoir*—until the *accouchement*." As I made my way down the stairs I thought of how I had felt the first time I went up them, and how much I had learned since then. It was like all the ads for dance studios or language records—"Learn to Whatever in Six Easy Lessons." But this time I was confident it was true. I had faith in Mme. Cohen and Dr. Lamaze, faith in Pavlov, and most of all faith in myself. I was looking forward to the championship match, confident that I would win. Not that I wanted to show off; but there was one face I did want to look into knowing I had done my best—the face of my child drawing his first breath.

5   La Méthode Lamaze

One spring day while we were browsing on the *quais*, I had come across a slightly used copy of a book by Colette Jeanson, *Principes et Pratique de l'Accouchement sans Douleur*. At last I was able to get the full story of the Pavlov method and of our busy and mysterious Dr. Lamaze.

The whole thing began, I discovered, not only with Pavlov, but with a whole series of attempts in Russia to make painless childbirth possible by the use of hypnosis. At first these attempts were purely experimental. But beginning in 1920 K. I. Platonov, A. P. Nicolaiev, and I. Z. Velvovski, began to investigate the physiologic bases of the action of hypnosis in childbirth. They based this work on the physiological studies that had already been done by Pavlov, and also on the studies of the physiology of hypnosis that Pavlov himself was engaged in at the same time. In the course of this work it was found desirable to supplement purely hypnotic techniques with a preliminary program of education of the expectant mother. Using this approach, a certain number of successful deliveries were performed. But the Russians were still not satisfied because of the difficulty of applying hypnotic techniques on a large scale. They found that the use of hypnosis was impracticable with large numbers of women and required exceptionally highly trained physicians to perform it successfully. What they were looking for was a method that would work equally well for everyone, and that could become widespread.

For this reason about 1930 hypnosis was definitely abandoned as a technique for the suppression of pain. The fact was that hypnosis was only a symptomatic medication for pain, and did not get at its causes. It was to the elucidation of the whole problem of pain in childbirth that the developers of what was later to be the psycho-prophylactic method now turned. Much of their work at this point was based on Pavlov's studies of the importance of what he called the "second system of signalization"—namely speech. By the process of trial and error a new method of painless childbirth based on the conscious education of women and the building up of consciously developed conditioned reflexes was evolved. It was tried out in clinics in Kharkov, Moscow and Leningrad. The results were so successful that in July of 1951 (following a recommendation of the Ministry of Public Health the previous February) a governmental decree generalized the method throughout the Soviet Union.

Later in the same summer Dr. Lamaze visited Professor Nicolaiev's clinic in Leningrad and saw the method in operation. On his return to France Dr. Lamaze immediately set about introducing the Russian method in the clinic of the metalworkers' union in Paris, whose lying-in section he directed. This naturally required a good deal of reorganization and training of personnel, but as early as May of 1952 most of the deliveries at the metalworkers' clinic were being performed by the psycho-prophylactic method. Nor was Dr. Lamaze content merely to accept the method as he had found it in Russia. He knew that it would have to be adapted to the French situation, and he and his associates were always alert for any improvements that could be made in practice. Much of this development was based on a careful study of the reports which every woman who had her child by this method was required to write shortly after her delivery. These reports were not supposed to be mere expressions of the woman's opinion, but rather a step-by-step description, as complete as possible, of everything she had felt and done during the delivery. The reports of the failures were even more eagerly studied than those of the successes, as it was hoped to eliminate causes of failure. I was fascinated to learn that the panting that Mme. Cohen had taught me, the blowing out during the period of transition, and much of the technique of pushing had been developed in France. It was also found possible to deliver breech babies and other less usual presentations more efficiently with the woman cooperating than with the woman anesthetized.

It did not take long for politics to get into the act. The French have an elaborate system of social security which pays many maternity costs. Moreover, the clinic of the metalworkers' union was already receiving a governmental subsidy to cover part of the difference between the rates paid by social security medical insurance and the cost of running the clinic. But the Pavlov method cost the clinic more than the conventional methods had, because it demanded more personnel and more space. So the clinic applied for a further subsidy, and the Pavlov method entered the political arena. It was, after all, imported from Russia, and the metalworkers' union was communist-dominated. Much of the debate that followed had little to do with medicine, but it did result in tremendous publicity for the method. A large section of Dr. Lamaze's private clientele deserted him. On the other hand, all over France people became interested, and *Accouchement sans Douleur* became a household word. (When Alex told our cleaning man that I had just had a baby, he was confronted with the unexpected question "*Avec ou sans douleur?*") *

Colette Jeanson's book also contained a theoretical discussion of the principles of Pavlovian physiology and obstetrics, that I, with my 68 in biology behind me, would not even attempt to reproduce. But it did fascinate me to learn of the many-sided attack the Pavlov method makes on pain. It led me to understand that none of the statements Mme. Cohen had made about pain was meant to sum up the entire Pavlov system. All of them were meant to complement each other.

The Pavlov method denies that pain is *essential* or beneficial to childbirth—which is not the same thing as saying that it does not exist or that it is an illusion. The Pavlov method, like all of medicine, is a mixture of the applications of biological theory and the results of purely empirical or experimental observations. Its understanding of pain and of how pain can be combatted is the same sort of mixture. The proof lies not in any theoretical logic, but rather in the fact that it works.

The first cause of pain recognized by the Pavlov method is fear, and the unfavorable reflexes fear creates. There is an absolute reflex that makes the body tense when a person becomes afraid.

---

* Dr. Lamaze's struggle to introduce *accouchement sans douleur* in France was the inspiration for a story that was later made into the film, *The Case of Dr. Laurent*, starring Jean Gabin, which has been widely shown in the United States and has met with highly enthusiastic critical reception. But the film is not, as one is tempted to assume, a fictionalized version of an actual incident in Dr. Lamaze's life, but a wholly original story that the writer Le Chamois was inspired to write by the adventure of *accouchement sans douleur* and the revolution in human relations he saw it working in France.

This reaction is reflected in the idiom "gripped by fear." Tense muscles, as Mme. Cohen pointed out, lead to pain. Furthermore, fear affects the brain adversely, and puts it in a condition in which any pain is experienced with greater intensity. The Pavlov method combats fear by education. It combats the tension caused by fear by creating conditioned reflexes of controlled relaxation which are able to overcome the defensive reflexes that lead to tension.

Another cause of pain related to the first is misinterpretation of sensation. Childbirth is a vigorous, active, muscular process. The contractions of the uterus, the moving of the baby down the birth canal, produce strong sensations, as does any vigorous muscular effort. A woman who is not prepared to experience these sensations, and knows nothing of what they are likely to be, will probably interpret them as pain. This interpretation will in turn lead to fear and even greater pain. This, too, is combatted by education.

Pain may also result from extraneous muscular interference with the action of the uterus. This the Pavlov method combats by the *effleurage* which relaxes the muscles of the abdominal wall, by chest breathing which keeps the pressure of the diaphragm on the uterus to a minimum, and by the techniques of controlled relaxation.

The pain of strong contractions may be caused by a lack of oxygen. This the Pavlov method combats by techniques of accelerated breathing and by giving additional oxygen between contractions whenever necessary.

During what are usually the two most difficult moments in childbirth (transition, crowning), pain is caused by the fact that the natural reflexes are ill-timed, that is, because the woman pushes when it would be better for her not to. The Pavlov method combats this pain by conditioning the pushing reflex so that the woman can control it and avoid pushing when the obstetrician tells her not to.

But in any particular case these methods for combatting pain may not work perfectly, and perhaps there is some other cause of pain, as yet unknown. So the Pavlov method attacks the residue of painful sensations by raising the sill of sensibility to a level where they are inhibited from entering consciousness. This is done by maintaining a high level of conscious activity throughout the delivery. The woman is warned to stay alert and to pay attention to everything that is happening to her; she constantly uses her brain to maintain control over her muscles. In this way all the techniques employed during the delivery, in addition to their direct effect on the muscles concerned, aid in the inhibition of the reception of pain in the cerebral cortex.*

At the back of Colette Jeanson's book, I found a number of the reports of women who had had babies by this method. I

---

* Two of Pavlov's experiments illustrate the mechanisms involved in painless childbirth. In the first, it is noted that when an electric shock is applied to a dog's paw, the dog has what is called a defense reflex—it barks, tries to get away, shows every sign of feeling pain, etc. For several days the electric shock is given simultaneously with food. It is noted that gradually the defense reflex becomes weaker and weaker. Finally the shock alone, without the food, produces not the defense reflex, but salivation with no sign of pain. A painful stimulus has been transformed into the signal for the salivary reflex. The British physiologist Sherrington when shown this experiment exclaimed, "Now I understand the psychology of martyrs."

The other experiment shows that pain can result from conditioning and be eliminated by conditioning in human beings, and that the spoken word can serve as the signal for both of these. A spiral tube is put about a man's arm; by sending water through it rapid and precise changes of temperature can be effected. It is noted that at 43 degrees Centigrade the man feels a pleasant warmth and the blood vessels of his arm dilate, while at 65 degrees he feels a painful heat and the blood vessels contract. When the 65-degree heat is applied a bell is rung. After a while the ringing of the bell *or the words* "I am going to ring" produces pain and contraction of the blood vessels even when the temperature applied is only 43 degrees. On the other hand the application of 65 degrees without ringing the bell and with the words "This is only warm" produces *no pain* and dilation instead of contraction of the blood vessels. More than that, when the region of the arm is anesthetized with novocaine, the painful degree of heat produces no pain or contraction, but the ringing of the bell continues to produce both.

read them avidly. I wanted to find out as much as possible about what I might expect from my own delivery. Any impression that I still had that the events would unroll in a simple, dull, over-scheduled manner was entirely banished. Each account read like an adventure. Every one of them reminded me that, while child-birth might be predicted with a great deal of accuracy, the events of the outside world—autos, subways, telephones, baby-sitters—would be as haphazard as ever, and that one's training might be put to the test of having to cope with any number of unanticipated occurrences. I admiringly read how each of these women had overcome every problem with courage and skill. Every one of them saw the *accouchement* as a series of challenges that she could and did confidently overcome. I was so impressed by the story of one woman who made a two-hour drive in a truck from the country to the hospital, controlling her contractions without anxiety, that I almost began to wish that I might be presented with some such test to try my skill. Reading the accounts of other women in their own words gave me a sense of the reality of the experience. I was determined to do as well as they.

The day arrived when we were to see the movie. We drove out to the *populaire* quarter of Menilmontant where, for the first time, we saw the clinic of the metalworkers' union. It stood facing a pleasant but noisy square, and once inside the gates, we came upon a scene of bustling activity. A great crowd of pregnant women, many of them accompanied by husbands and even children, was pouring into a large hall. I was astonished at the idea that any one doctor could have so many patients. As it turned out, Dr. Lamaze was assisted by his associate, Dr. Vellay, and several other doctors. Now a technician was running up and down the aisle trying to adjust the sixteen-millimeter projector so that the picture approximated the size of the small screen that stood at one end of the hall. The scene had that casual, homey atmosphere that I associate with the presentation of amateur movies. I half expected to see shots of the activities at the last season of the union camp. I suppose I was led to that idea by the number of enthusiastic little children who ran happily up and down the aisles, crawling in and out over the rows of chairs.

Suddenly a door opened and Dr. Lamaze came in to introduce the film. There was an immediate respectful hush. He spoke in the same friendly humorous manner that he had in his office. The film we were about to see, he explained, had been put together from various sources and some parts of it were very old. He told us briefly what it contained so that we would have no difficulty in following it. As he finished the lights flicked off and the show began.

The first part showed some pictures of Pavlov followed by some scenes that looked like a nursery school—it was hard to tell if Pavlov was directing the children or not, and I missed whatever the point of the goings-on was. Then suddenly there was a horror sequence that showed a very old-fashioned delivery. The woman was obviously making a terrible racket as she leapt up and down like an epileptic. The nurses were holding her down while the doctor engaged in what looked like a tug of war. It was a nightmare. I looked to see what kind of a traumatic effect it was having on the children in the audience, but they were merely looking around them with expressions of unconcern. Two of them were rolling a ball up and down the aisle. They didn't appear to understand or care about what was going on—fortunately, I thought. The scene left me feeling somewhat sick, and a little rebellious at what was obviously the beginning of a hard sell.

The next sequence moved into more familiar territory—young women in a classroom listening to a lecture. Then the same young women were shown lying on tables, doing the same exercises I had learned—and then a scene of a young woman having a baby and smiling. In contrast with the previous delivery, this one was obviously taking place in an atmosphere of peace and happiness. The people in the delivery room moved very little and appeared to do very little talking as well. The woman on the table had an expression of intense concentration, which her attendants gave every indication of respecting. As the period of expulsion went on she seemed to be working very hard, but between the contractions she was relaxed and peaceful. The doctor delivered the baby very slowly.

When I saw what it looked like as the head crowned, I was terror stricken. It seemed the head couldn't possibly get through without tearing her to shreds. I wasn't the only one who was worried. There was a great gasp from the audience. Only the people on the screen seemed free from anxiety. Slowly, gently, the head was worked out, and when the face was turned up so that you could see the features there was a terrible sigh of relief. Then the doctor in the film turned the head in his hands and deftly extracted the baby's right arm which he placed on the mother's thigh. At that moment she looked up into the face of her baby, and the expression on her face was radiant. The doctor turned the baby again, and then all at once he lifted him out and up into the air for the mother to admire. At this point, even some of the children in the audience began to pay attention and to join in the "ohs" and "ahs" of delight at the new little child.

Then before I had time to decide whether I found the scene frightening or reassuring, another delivery took place, giving us an opportunity to witness the entire miracle all over again from the very start. The second time I paid even more attention to the actual delivery of the baby's head. I found it difficult to believe that the head could really be born without the most excruciating agony and destruction, and even as I watched it going on in front of my eyes, I was still obsessed by the notion that it was an impossibility. It was reassuring to see that birth was feasible, and how short a time the freeing of the head really took. The mother's face was truly beautiful. I had become so absorbed in the delivery of the head that I had failed to observe what the mother herself had been doing. On later reflection I decided that that was not the purpose of the film at all, and that it had actually performed the function that had been intended for me.

As I stood up to leave I found that my knees were trembling; something in me had been deeply shocked. I took Alex's arm for support and stumbled along to the nearest café. We both ordered double cognacs—for medicinal purposes, Alex said.

"They really oughtn't to show such things," I began. "Traumatic! Can only create fear." But even as I said it I began to feel calm. So that was what it was to have a child. Actually it was very simple. Simple and human; nothing mysterious—only the mystery of birth itself. And everyone looking so calm and happy.

As it happened the film turned out to have been a wonderful psychological experience. As the days went by I thought over those scenes again and again, visualizing them, trying to digest what I had seen and to come to terms with it. I found that my sense of shock faded away bit by bit, and was replaced by that happy sense of security that attaches to familiar things. It seemed unlikely that I could be twice shocked by the same thing, and I began to be confident that when it was my turn to deliver I would remember what I had seen, and know that there was nothing to fear. As for the first sequence, when I thought it over I realized that it was just some such scene that had previously been somewhere in the back of my mind, associated with the word childbirth. I was glad that it too had been brought out in the open where I could look at it, and that I had been shown the movie far enough in advance for that process of digestion to take place. It was one of the most helpful parts of the education.

A few days after the movie, I went alone to take the hospital tour. By that time I felt I could face anything, and I drove up to the hospital with a feeling of real anticipation. It was such a pleasant place. There were several other girls waiting when I arrived. We were left in the salon, a large room in the center of the ground floor with French doors opening out onto the back garden. It was pleasantly cool and quiet there, a relief after the long drive through traffic. We wandered aimlessly about as if we were waiting for nothing in particular. Soon there were seventeen of us, all curiously silent and shy.

Suddenly a conversation began. It was carried on in subdued tones between a very young girl having her first child and a much older woman about to have her fifth. It would have been an argument except that the two of them were in essential agreement about the main point—that it was impossible that one could really have a child without suffering excruciating anguish. The young girl kept repeating nervously that no matter what anyone told her, she *knew* that having children gave you palpitations of the heart. The elegant older woman replied that she doubted that very seriously, although she was certain that there couldn't be such a thing as painless childbirth. She had gone through torture during her first four deliveries; she was in a position to know. Of course she hadn't tried this way before, but after all! The two of them sniped at each other intermittently. The rest of us were silent. From time to time we all sneaked oblique glances at each other's maternity dresses. My American clothes were comparatively chic, since the *haute couture* of France hadn't really buckled down to the problems of the pregnant woman. But none of us was ravishing.

At last a great blond nurse came to announce that we were all invited to go home. The hospital was full, there were no vacant delivery rooms to snoop about in, and besides she didn't see the use of such nonsense. But because we had all come such a long distance, because it was such a very hot day, and more especially because this was France, no one stirred a step. The nurse stood looking at us with disgust for a few seconds and then went away muttering. When another fifteen minutes had gone by she returned still scowling. There was another nurse right behind her. I wondered if we were about to be forcibly evicted. The second nurse smiled at us pleasantly. "You understand how it is with nature," she began. "Babies don't wait . . ." We stared impassively. *We* could wait.

"Well," she said, "if you insist on staying—there is one of Dr. Lamaze's patients who is in the smallest delivery room. [At the Belvédère you stayed in the same room throughout labor and delivery.] She is having a premature birth—seven months, so she hasn't yet begun to train." We stared silently. The blond nurse sputtered out something that sounded like "*Imbéciles!*" The second nurse shrugged her shoulders. She had the good sense to see that she was licked. "You may come along then," she said. "The *monitrice* is with her, teaching as they go, and though I don't recommend it, she doesn't mind if you come—only please, just eight at a time. The room is so small." I was appalled. "I wouldn't like this crew to troop in on *me*," I thought. But I went along with the others.

We straggled along, down the hall, through the door that warned all extraneous people to keep out, and there we were in the modern delivery wing. The blond nurse came trailing along after us, still muttering imprecations and doing her best to make us feel like the guilty intruders we were about to be. Finally the first group tiptoed into the small delivery room, leaving the rest of us to wait interminably in the corridor. When at last they had tiptoed out again, we stealthily moved to take their places. After all that build-up I expected to see something really dramatic. I was disappointed.

It was a small room. There was a bed, a table, a chair, an oxygen tank and a little cabinet full of bedpans. I was vaguely disturbed. Where were the medical things in case of emergency? In another room, I was told; emergencies are not so common. The young woman on the bed looked over at us and smiled. She said she felt just fine. The nervous girl immediately asked her if she wasn't having some palpitations.

"No, not at all," the imminent mother began. But suddenly she stopped, looked off into space and began to pant. The *monitrice* stood beside her and panted right along to keep her company. We stared, fascinated. "Stop now," said the *monitrice*, exhaling a long slow breath. She stopped and turned back to us. "Where were we?" she asked. "Oh yes, palpitations . . ."

"But isn't she having advanced-stage contractions?" someone asked. "Doesn't that panting come toward the end?"

"Yes," the *monitrice* smiled, "we are doing very nicely."

Someone else asked to see the stirrups that would be used during the period of expelling the baby. The young girl began to pant again, and as soon as she had finished the contraction, she moved over to allow the *monitrice* to demonstrate the stirrups to her audience. We stood there, huddled together at an acceptable distance, and stared about for a few more minutes, baffled by the evident simplicity of the room and the labor that was in progress. Then we thanked the two of them for their hospitality and filed out much more noisily than we had entered. The visit had begun by showing all the signs of being a fiasco, but it had turned out to be even more profitable than I had anticipated. It was a good thing to become acquainted with the delivery room, but to see it while it was in use was much, much better. It was becoming obvious that the closer one came to the facts of childbirth, the less frightening they seemed.

"Now," our guide said when we were out in the corridor, "we are going to visit a young woman who had her baby last week." In we trooped, this time to a large and pleasantly furnished corner room. At one side, in a bassinet draped with pink and white ribbons, was the baby—her first. How miraculous! The nervous young girl looked over uncomfortably at the baby and began her questions again. "Did you do this? Did you feel that? Was it terrible?" All the answers were the same; "Oh, no, it was wonderful!" Then the elegant lady suggested that perhaps she had already forgotten the suffering—the memory is likely to repress such things. But already she looked beaten.

One by one the other girls found their tongues and pretty soon the poor mother was drenched in questions. She answered each one patiently, explaining her sensations at each and every moment, what techniques she had used, and how successful they had proved. She particularly insisted that the expulsion, far from being the worst phase, was absolutely painless and so very thrilling that she would happily do it again tomorrow. At this everyone became terribly enthusiastic, and began to exchange stories about other people who had had painless childbirth. There was a great deal of noise, with everyone talking at once in the way that only women have mastered to perfection. A nurse came running in to tell us that we were disturbing the peace of the establishment, and our guide whisked us out and down the hall for our next visit.

The second visit was even more startling than the first. This young woman was also a first-time mother. She had come to the hospital the evening before and had delivered early that very morning. She looked a little tired, but very pleased with herself and her baby. Her testimony dismissed any doubts that could possibly have remained in my head.

With these visits my proselytization was complete. The only thing that could now influence my feelings about the Pavlov method would be the success or failure of my own delivery. I couldn't imagine that it would be anything but a success. I think the others must have felt the same. We were a transformed group of women, and we rushed out of the hospital chattering enthusiastically, eager for the time when we could return to try it for ourselves.

My last visit to Dr. Lamaze gave an additional boost to my confidence. He inquired about my progress with Mme. Cohen, and seemed satisfied by my answers to the questions he asked me about the course. During my examination, he explained to me the position that the baby was in and assured me that it was the most auspicious position possible. My condition in general he described as admirable, and in order to keep it that way for the remaining two weeks, he prescribed a cream that would prevent the formation of any stretch marks on the abdomen. I asked him if this was part of the Pavlov method. "No," he answered with a smile, "it's part of staying a beautiful woman." I was delighted to find that with everything else he had to attend to he still took the time to pay attention to this.

"*Madame, vous êtes parfaite!*" he pronounced as I stood up. "I hope that the next time I see you will be at the Belvédère. Mme. Cohen will review you on the signs of labor. At the first one do not hesitate to call me—no matter what awkward time of day or night it is. You or your husband will telephone me, and I will tell you when to present yourself at the clinic. You need worry about nothing else but getting there. I will tell them to expect you. I will reach Mme. Cohen for you. I know that you will be too excited at the beginning of labor to want to worry about details. So leave them all to me. And now, madame, *bon chance!*"

My last lesson with Mme. Cohen had been on June 30. The baby was scheduled to arrive on the fifth of July. On the third we drove to Chartres for the day. I was afraid that we wouldn't have another chance for an outing for some time, and I wanted to cram in as much as possible before we had definitively entered the category of parents. On the evening of the fourth we went to a very late cocktail party. On the morning of the fifth I got up and waited for the baby. The fifth passed and then the sixth. Neither of us was able to work or study. We began to recalculate the day of arrival. I read and reread Colette Jeanson's book and practiced every day so as to stay as conditioned as possible. More days went by. I called Mme. Cohen and she made another appointment for me to come in and rehearse. It was important for me to keep up my conditioning.

I found it more and more difficult to pass by those marvelous shops full of baby clothes without buying anything. There was one little dress in particular that I developed a powerful craving for. I had a strong intuition that the baby was going to turn out to be a girl. It was followed up by another strong intuition to the effect that she would be born on the fourteenth. We agreed that we would call her Marianne in honor of the French Republic. I had heard that the government gave special bonuses for children born on the fourteenth. As far as I was concerned it was all settled.

On the morning of the fourteenth I got out my suitcase and put it in the trunk of the car. We walked up and down the quays half the day; in the evening we went to the *bal* on the prow of the Ile-Saint-Louis and danced happily until midnight. The fourteenth had passed and there was still no baby. I began to think that the entire thing was an illusion; there was no baby. The next day I was in a terrible temper. I refused to practice my exercises. I insisted that we go to the Méditerranée for lunch, and I packed away everything from bouillabaisse to chocolate soufflé. I don't remember how I managed to get through the afternoon. At dinnertime I ate again with a vengeance. I was in that terrible state of nerves that is inevitable when you have successfully got through the dress rehearsal, but you don't know when you will be able to hold the opening night.

We saw on a poster that several rooms at the Louvre were going to be illuminated that evening. Immediately after coffee we drove over and wandered about the exhibit of Roman sculpture. There we distracted each other by making unpleasant comments about the emperors from Augustus downhill. I was particularly pleased to discover that Caligula looked just like a modern American juvenile delinquent. We met some New York friends alongside a bust of Agrippina, and all went on together to the Flore where we discussed painting till after one o'clock in the morning. By this time I was so bitter that I didn't care what was going on. We arrived home at nearly two in the morning. I was tired and discouraged. I undressed and got into bed, resigned to the fact that the baby would never arrive.

The minute I turned out the light a contraction began. I leapt up and looked at the clock. We waited. Ten minutes later there was another.

"What do we do now?" Alex asked.

"Time them a little longer," I said.

We waited together in silence, watching the clock. It was ludicrous. The hands moved terribly slowly. Then, sure enough, exactly ten minutes later, another contraction.

"I think I'll call Dr. Lamaze," Alex said. He grabbed some change and rushed out to the *tabac*. Two minutes later he was back again. "He says to wait until the contractions come every seven minutes, then call him again and go to the hospital." We looked at the clock for another hour. The contractions were coming regularly every seven or eight minutes. I picked up my toothbrush and we left.

The *tabac* had closed. We drove to the Café du Dôme in Montparnasse and telephoned from there. The night was fresh and full of the smell of earth that blows over Paris on summer nights. "Come ahead," Dr. Lamaze said. We stopped to put down the top of the car, and then we drove to the hospital. The city was beautiful and still as we drove along; it was a perfect night to have a baby.

6　C'est Un Garçon!

When we arrived at four A.M., the whole hospital was dark except for the front hall. A nurse was waiting for us—what efficiency for Paris! She led the way to the delivery room, and

Alex followed us with the suitcase. He put it down on a stand in the corner of the room, and we stood looking at each other, wondering what to do next. The contractions were coming regularly every seven minutes, but they were very weak and didn't require any action on my part at all. As we stood there waiting, I felt another one. It was an interesting sensation, rather like the way it feels when you flex the muscle of your calf, but it didn't even seem worth sitting down for. I was very excited, thoroughly alert, and there was nothing to do. When the nurse came back, I looked to her for suggestions.

"Get out the clothes," she directed. Alex opened the suitcase, and I began to sort through the things I had put there, what seemed to be ages ago, wondering just what was the right thing to *accouche* in. "I don't want those," the nurse interrupted when she saw what I was doing. "The baby clothes!"

So there *was* going to be a real baby! The nurse went to the suitcase herself, and we watched her pick out the things she wanted and arrange them neatly on a table, all ready to receive little Marianne or Pepi, whenever she or he (I was still certain it would be she) made up her mind to put in an appearance. For all the months of anticipation and planning we had been through, I think that was the first moment that Alex or I really believed in the existence of the baby.

Before she went out again, the nurse pulled a short nightgown out of my suitcase and indicated that that was what I was to wear. As there was only one chair in the room, and Alex looked tired, I decided to get into bed to wait for things to start happening. A few minutes later a midwife came in and examined me. "Very little dilatation," she said. "Certainly not before nine in the morning. Probably not before noon."

She went out. We sat and talked for a while. Outside the city was very still. Alex began to yawn, and finally decided that as nothing was going to happen for a few hours, he might as well go home and get a little sleep. I supposed I ought to sleep too.

The contractions were regular but still very weak, and Mme. Cohen had stressed the importance of rest before the delivery. Almost before Alex had shut the door behind him, I was off in a deep sleep. I hadn't realized how the past few days had exhausted me.

Sunlight was pouring in the window when I was awakened again by the increased force of the contractions. I looked at my watch and timed a few. They were coming regularly every five minutes, and they lasted nearly fifty seconds. They felt like the earlier ones, only stronger, with now and then a suggestion, or maybe only the threat, of a cramp. I found that by merely relaxing and doing the slow, deep breathing, they remained in the category of interesting muscular sensations. Nothing more. I didn't see any reason to begin the *effleurage*. The only thing that bothered me was the possibility that they might suddenly get stronger before Alex got back to the hospital. This idea kept me looking anxiously from my watch to the door.

At nine o'clock a new midwife came in to ask how I felt. Was I perfectly comfortable? I said that I was, but she still walked about the table puffing up the pillows under my head, and put a bolster under my knees to make sure that I was perfectly relaxed. She went out, promising to send in a nurse with some tea, and to come back again to see how I was getting along. I hoped she would hurry, because I was very curious to know how I was doing.

No sooner had I finished my tea, than the midwife was back again. She carefully pushed away the *traversin* she had so recently adjusted, and examined me very gently. "Well?" I asked. "Soon?"

"Is this your first?" she said in a tone that indicated that she was pretty sure it was. I nodded. "Be patient," she smiled. "Not before four in the afternoon."

"But how can that be?" I asked. "How far is the dilatation?"

In answer she showed me the tip of her forefinger. Practically nothing. I was disappointed. What on earth had been happening for all those hours? I waited, breathing slowly from the beginning of each contraction. I was terribly bored. I could feel the contractions gathering force and growing stronger. I tried out the *effleurage*, but it didn't really seem necessary. A nurse came in and put some things in the sterilizer. She looked at me thoughtfully and smiled. "You look bored," she said. "Why don't you go out for a nice walk in the garden?"

"But I don't want to walk in the garden," I said. I explained to her that the dilatation was only about the size of the tip of my forefinger, and that I was becoming discouraged. She insisted more than ever that what I really needed was a nice walk in the fresh air. "How often do you have contractions?" she asked.

"Every five minutes."

She looked at me skeptically, shrugged her shoulders and disappeared. I sat up and began to wonder where my bathrobe and slippers were. I found them, got up, and went to the sink to rinse my mouth. But at that moment the contractions became stronger, and I decided to forgo the walk in the garden, and got back in bed. The contractions kept coming and coming. I kept doing the slow breathing, concentrating on each one to learn all I could about it. If the cervix wasn't doing its part, at least I was doing mine.

Then, somehow, I drifted off to sleep. That was when I got my first practical lesson on how very important it is to stay awake. I couldn't have been sleeping long when I awoke in a kind of nightmare of throbbing pain. I tried to remember to breathe, but before I could catch up with the contraction, it stopped, and I dozed off again. This must have happened several times. The pain I felt was like the cramp you get in your side when you run right after a heavy meal. It couldn't have been very strong, because the moment it stopped I dozed off to sleep again. (I had had no drugs. I was just tired.) Fortunately Alex was there, and he soon realized what was happening. He woke me up by sponging my face with cold water, and told me to begin the rapid breathing. As soon as I was awake again, I regained my control, and the pain vanished. Alex checked my arms and legs to see that I was relaxed. I tried to go back to the slow breathing, but I found that its usefulness was past.

That was at two in the afternoon. From time to time I was examined by different midwives. They all had the same story to tell—very little progress in the dilatation. The contractions were somewhat stronger. They were coming every four minutes. I was still in control. I could sense the threat of pain under the muscular effort of my uterus, but as long as I did the breathing and the *effleurage* it was only a threat. All the same, I was tired and beginning to be discouraged. I very much regretted all the follies of the past week. Despite all the warnings I had received, I had come to my *accouchement* in a state of general fatigue. Now that I saw that it was going to be a long, demanding affair, I wondered if I really would have the energy I needed to stay in control until the end. I was miserable at the thought that I might not see the birth of my child.

The afternoon was coming to an end. The midwives had stopped making time predictions. The daylight gradually faded, the sound of children's voices playing in a soccer field near the clinic stopped, and a drowsy calm came over me. The room slowly grew dim. I stopped thinking of anything but contractions. I had become a mechanism that concentrated, breathed rhythmically, relaxed, and performed an abstract hand movement known as *effleurage*. I wasn't even discouraged. It was all very businesslike, only tedious.

A nurse brought me some mashed potatoes and another cup of tea. I gobbled it down between contractions, and then wished there was more. Eating revived me. I felt less tired. Alex found that he was hungry too, and went out to look for a sandwich. A midwife came in and examined me. I continued my breathing right through the examination. Then she went out and returned with another midwife who also examined me. I looked at them and became interested in something outside my contractions.

They had retired to a corner of the room for a whispered conversation. I listened intently, trying to pick out any words I could. Did I hear the word "Cesarian," or just something else in French that sounded like that? Then they went out together absorbed in an argument that I supposed could only concern me.

A minute or so later a nurse I hadn't seen before marched briskly into the room, and before I could say anything she injected a hypo of something into me. I remember feeling terribly confused and distressed. Then, before I realized what had happened to me, I dropped off into a state of semi-sleep and a recurrent nightmare of pain.

Alex came back and did what he could to help me. He washed my face and tried to tell me when to breathe, but the effect of whatever it was I had been given was too strong. I kept dozing off between contractions, and waking only when they were already under way. Mme. Cohen's analogy of the wave proved only too true. No matter how hard I tried, fighting against the contraction and the effect of the drug on my brain all at once was too much; I could not regain my control. The pain I felt was similar to that I had felt the last time I fell asleep; only now it was stronger and instead of throbbing it rose to a peak along with the contraction. I could truly imagine that if it got much worse, it would be unbearable. How I regretted not being in the metalworkers' clinic where *all* the personnel were trained in the principles of the method and a mistake like that of giving me a hypo would not have occurred!

The midwife came back and examined me. This time she had good news. The dilatation was nearly at five francs. At last the contractions were doing their work. But I remained discouraged. I was sure that if things went on the way they were going, I would have to be put out before the end. I even had a moment of real doubt about the whole Pavlov method, and wondered if contractions didn't *have* to be painful before they did any good.

This time it was Mme. Cohen who saved me. She appeared in

the doorway, all fresh and sparkling, took in the situation at a glance, and set about restoring my control. Her first move was to turn on all the lights, instead of just the little night light that had been on till then. She bathed my face and neck with cold water until I was thoroughly awake, and commanded me to breathe and relax. By that time I had to be told; I was still too sleepy to judge for myself. I couldn't manage to recognize the beginning of a contraction. Mme. Cohen put Alex to work sponging my face with cold water, while she directed my breathing and *effleurage* with one hand on my stomach. She was able to recognize the beginning of a contraction before I did, and she breathed along with me, stopping when it had passed its peak, so that all I had to do was imitate her. Between contractions she made sure I was totally relaxed. In a few minutes the pain stopped and my control returned. The contractions regained shape and form, and I was able to stay on top of them.

But there was very little time in between, and I was exhausted. Mme. Cohen sent for a glucose injection that, she explained, would give me the energy I needed for the expulsion.* At the very sound of the word "expulsion" my confidence returned. The next examination showed that I had passed five francs. At last, I was making progress. I was sure the baby would be born before long, and that I would be fully conscious when it was.

Dr. Lamaze arrived. He examined me carefully, and seemed entirely satisfied with my progress. By that time I was no longer talking to anyone, not even to him. I was much too busy. I didn't look at my watch again until after the delivery was over. Mme. Cohen gave me some oxygen with the plexiglass mask. I remember being surprised that it didn't have any smell or taste, and I was not able to judge its effect. The contractions had become very strong. It took all my concentration, even with Mme. Cohen directing me, to remain in control. For a while it seemed that the

---

* In some cases certain obstetricians also employ coramine-glucose, a heart and respiratory stimulant.

contractions merged into one, but Mme. Cohen kept telling me when to breathe and when to rest. Looking back on it now, I see that it was the hardest work I had ever done in my life, just as Mme. Cohen said it would be.

I remember the moment when the transition period began very clearly. For no apparent reason, I suddenly stopped breathing. My only sensation was one of extreme nervousness. For a moment I didn't know what was happening. Then I concluded that I must be experiencing a desire to push, although I couldn't exactly say that I really felt like pushing. What I really felt was a desire to do nothing at all. After a moment of that suspended state, the desire to push suddenly came on me overwhelmingly. "*Ça vient!*" I shouted.

"*Pas encore,*" Mme. Cohen said. There was an immediate scurry of activity all about me. Dr. Lamaze adjusted a light, Mme. Cohen removed all my pillows, and a midwife and nurse arranged my feet in the stirrups. "*Pas encore,*" Mme. Cohen repeated several times. I panted and puffed and blew, and waited for the word to come. It was an unbelievable sensation, not at all painful but somewhat terrifying.

Finally Mme. Cohen told me I could push. What a relief! No matter what I had imagined about pushing during my rehearsals, I was tremendously surprised by what a satisfying sensation it was. Dr. Lamaze called the signals—"*Inspirez! Soufflez! Inspirez! Bloquez! Poussez!*—and I performed automatically, just as Mme. Cohen said I would during the first lesson when she explained conditioned reflexes. (It must have been automatic because Alex told me later I did just what I was told, and I don't remember thinking of what to do.) But there was a new element I had not expected. From the moment I began to push, the atmosphere of the delivery room underwent a radical transformation. Where previously everyone had spoken in soft and moderate tones in deference to my state of concentration, now there was a wild encouraging cheering section, dedicated to spurring me on. I felt like a football star, headed for a touchdown. My fans on the sidelines, Dr. Lamaze, Mme. Cohen, the midwife, the nurse, all exhorted me, "*POUSSEZ! POUSSEZ! POUSSEZ! POUSSEZ! CONTINUEZ! CONTINUEZ! CONTINUEZ! ENCORE! ENCORE!*" When I ran out of breath, Mme. Cohen reminded me to exhale, inhale, and hold again. When the contraction was over, the cheering stopped. Each time a new contraction began and I started to push again, the cheering section burst forth. It was fantastically exhilarating; it made me push harder and harder. Then, finally (Alex says the pushing took twenty minutes), the head crowned.

"*Ne poussez plus, madame!*"

This time it was very easy. I lay back, relaxed, and began to pant. But suddenly a sharp pain shot through my left leg. I winced and turned to Mme. Cohen. "Relax your leg," she said.

"I can't."

"You have a muscle cramp." She massaged it deftly, and in a few seconds it was gone. The minute my leg stopped hurting I became aware of a sensation that momentarily horrified me. Dr. Lamaze was working at turning down the baby's head, and I could feel everything he was doing! I had no sensation of pain at all, but I was shocked by the fact that my perception of what was happening was so complete. I felt the presence of the head, but I felt it the way I had felt the existence of a hole the dentist was drilling in my novocained tooth, touching it with my tongue. It seemed immense! Frighteningly so.

At that moment the delivery sequence of the movie flashed into my mind. I saw the doctor working the head down—just as Dr. Lamaze was doing at that minute. I knew there was nothing to be frightened of. I continued to pant, watching the delivery in my mind as it progressed.

"Forehead, eyes, nose . . ." I heard Dr. Lamaze call out slowly. "Come here, monsieur, come quickly! *Venez voir votre enfant naître!*—Come see your child is born!"

For an instant I thought of reminding Alex of his promise to stay at the head of the bed, but then I heard a tiny cry "La!" and realized how absurd I was. I felt something hot and wet on my leg. It was the baby's arm. Everyone shouted "Look!" Mme. Cohen helped me to raise my head and shoulders, and there I was looking into the face of my baby who was crying sweetly before he was completely born. A second more and Dr. Lamaze held him up for me to see. "*C'est un garçon, madame*," he announced. He placed him on a sheet over my stomach so that I could hold him for a moment. It was incredible—he had my father's eyes, a Karmel forehead, and a cleft chin like Alex's, and yet he was obviously a real individual in his own right, from the very first moment. We named him immediately, Joseph Low, after my father. We even settled on the nickname "Pepi."

After we had admired him properly, Dr. Lamaze cut the cord and handed him to a nurse who took him off to the corner to be washed and dressed in the clothes that had been waiting for so long. It was twenty minutes past two, July the seventeenth, over twenty-four hours since I had felt the first contraction. I had forgotten all about the placenta, but Mme. Cohen reminded me to push when the contraction came, and I expelled it easily. Everyone examined it, including me; then all of them but Alex tidied up and went away. The baby, all dressed and wrapped in a blanket, French style, was in a little cradle beside my bed. Alex and I were alone with him. It was less than fifteen minutes after he had been born.

We sat and listened to the baby gurgle and hiccup in the quiet of the warm, still night. As it was so late, I was not going to be moved to my room until the morning. In spite of the tremendous exertion I had been through, I felt wonderfully exhilarated and excited. We talked quietly about the delivery and about our plans for the future, but mainly we were just happy to be there together with our newborn child. Finally Alex went off to send telegrams.

I turned off the light, but for a long time I could not sleep. I lay in the dark and listened to the little noises my baby made and felt as happy as I had ever been.

A week later my mother flew over to see her grandchild. She was delighted with him and astonished at how alert he was and how his eyes seemed to look right at her without wandering around. At first I thought this was just standard grandmotherly exaggeration, but she insisted that most newborn babies she had ever seen looked like they were drunk for several weeks. I asked Dr. Lamaze about this, when he paid me a visit, and he told me that many of the effects my mother had described were caused by anesthesia and the added time the baby spent in the birth canal in a "normal" delivery.

My mother was thoroughly incredulous when I told her about the Pavlov method, and my experience. But when I really went into it, she admitted there might be something to it. Then, for the first time in our lives, we discussed the subject of childbirth. And for the first time, I realized why she had never spoken of it before. My recollection that my father had once mentioned finding her alone in a pool of blood was substantiated. And other details, no less horrifying, were added. This had all happened in one of the best hospitals in the capital of the United States not so very long ago. She looked back on her experience with childbirth as an ordeal that had been necessary, but certainly not as something to talk about. I couldn't help marveling at the difference between her feelings and mine. I was thankful that her fundamental tact had kept me from being conditioned in a way that might have been difficult to overcome, and I was even more thankful that a series of happy chances had led me to Dr. Lamaze and an experience that I would be proud and happy to tell to *my* children.

7 *In Search of a Doctor*

When we landed in New York a few months later the news of our exciting adventure had already fanned out ahead of us. The members of our families and friends who came to meet us had scarcely paid their proper respects to Pepi when someone asked Alex with an expression that was half questioning frown and half leer, "So! Were you really there when he made his first appearance?"

Alex assured him he was.

"You weren't there the *whole* time?"

"The *whole* time," Alex said.

"It must have been a horrible experience," someone commiserated, patting him sympathetically on the shoulder.

"No," said Alex, "it was inspiring."

One tactful old lady waited until we were alone to speak. "Well, my dear," she began hesitantly, "so they didn't give you anything for it." I assumed she was referring to drugs.

"That's right," I agreed. "Nothing at all."

"That's the way it is over there," she nodded. "Backward. Haven't made any scientific advancement. Not living in the modern world. That's the way it used to be. Now in America they can—"

"No, really," I interrupted, "I wanted it that way."

"Of course." She squinted at me suspiciously. "But would you go through it again?"

"I intend to. Yes."

Suddenly she drew herself up straight. She looked at me triumphantly. "There you are!" she said. "That's exactly what I think. In my day people didn't make such a fuss about having children. That's what a woman is made for, isn't it? Suffering is part of living. People are spoiled now . . . they pamper themselves! I had five children and nobody ever gave *me* anything. It's worth the pain. Better for the child. But don't listen to me. Nobody ever does."

Obviously there was no reason to pursue the discussion. In her mind there were only two possibilities—pain or drugs. Of the two, she preferred pain. It was part of her experience. Very likely she was heartily sick of hearing about the superiority of the modern world over that of her youth. In some way my experience vindicated her. I could see I had made her tremendously happy. "God bless you," she muttered several times, and as she left she kissed me—for the first time in many years.

I didn't find that reaction terribly hard to understand. But many of the others I encountered in the course of the next few months seemed extraordinarily incomprehensible. Before my first pregnancy I had never given any thought at all to the question of how to have a baby; I can't remember ever having heard it discussed at all, beyond the most minimal attention given it in a college hygiene course where it was almost totally eclipsed by the much more interesting question of how to conceive a baby. Therefore the discovery of the vast quantity of intensely felt convictions and prejudices that exist on the subject came to me as something of a revelation. Now an accident of fate had not only made me familiar with the facts of childbirth, but had taught me an effective and rewarding way to cope with them. I was delighted by the discovery I had made. So delighted, in fact, that it had never once crossed my mind that anyone else might fail to find it equally delightful.

I was still in this sweet state of innocence when one of my oldest friends invited us to a dinner party. It promised to be a relaxed informal evening. As things turned out, it was relaxed and pleasant through about the second round of cocktails. Suddenly, without any warning, cocktail shaker in hand, our host, Bob, said to Alex, "What is this stuff I've been hearing about your going in for obstetrics?"

We were off. We gave them a short version of our Paris adventure—short not from any lack of enthusiasm, but because we were hungry, and we could smell the dinner cooking. As I neared the end of the tale, I noticed that a girl we had just met for the first time was staring at me with a hostility she took no pains to conceal.

"You must have been hypnotized," she interrupted flatly. She wasn't going to be taken in by anything.

"Now Ronnie," her husband said in a conciliating tone, "you have no basis for such an assumption. After all you can be practically certain that primitive woman—"

Fortunately he never got to finish that flattering comparison.

"I'm sure it works if you believe in it," our hostess cut in quickly. "And if you think it's worth the trouble. When you've had four children as I have you'll probably look at it all in a different light. I used to be the way you are. I even had rooming-in with the first. Never again."

"That's not the same question, dear," Bob interrupted her.

"It's all the same thing," she said. "I adore my obstetrician. I go to the hospital and he puts me out. I don't want to know anything about it. I wake up after it's all over. The baby is in the nursery. I take a look at it and go back to sleep. I never feel anything. I don't love my children any the less for it. Probably, if you could measure it, you'd find I love them a little more."

"Shelley can't tolerate pain, you know," Bob explained, "and I don't see any reason why she should have to."

"Of course not," I agreed. "But that's just the point of the Pavlov method. There isn't any pain—"

"Not for you," said a friend of mine who had just had her first child. "Let's qualify that statement. Some of us are braver than others."

"What!" I exclaimed. "How can you say that? You know what a coward I am about the dentist!"

"The dentist is another matter. You have sensitive teeth. That's all that proves. But you have short, easy labors. Now in my case it would be out of the question. Actually, I'd like to have natural childbirth, but if you went through fourteen hours of torture as I did—"

"Fourteen! I was in labor for twenty-four!"

"Without taking anything? You must have no nervous system."

"No, really," I insisted, "I couldn't have done it if I hadn't known what to do."

"You'll never convince me," she said, shaking her head. "I know what it's like. I've been through it. I *know* I couldn't bear it without anesthesia. There's no point even talking about it."

In spite of myself, I began to get angry.

"So!" I said. "You had anesthesia? The purpose of which is to spare you pain?"

"That's right."

"Then how does it happen that you know so much about how terrible it was? What kind of anesthesia was that?"

"Twilight sleep."

"It sounds like pretty painful sleep," I said.

"Well," she reflected, "it's not really sleep so much as a twilight nightmare. But I prefer it that way."

"Fine," I said. "Let's change the subject. The men look bored to death."

"By no means," said Gloria's husband. "You girls never cease to fascinate me."

We all looked at him suspiciously for a moment. Then Gloria couldn't restrain herself. "I never thought you would turn into a martyr," she said. "It's not your style at all."

"But I'm not a martyr!" I repeated. I felt like one now.

"No, honestly," Shelley said, "I agree with the education part. One ought to know and that sort of thing. And certainly it's a good idea to relax—if you have the time to do exercises. But I know it wouldn't work for me . . . If I relaxed I would still suffer, and I'm squeamish about blood and such things."

"Something's burning," said Bob.

We went in to dinner.

"You know, Shelley, you remind me of a book I read somewhere, or was it in a magazine," Gloria said as she took her place at the table. "Well, anyway, the point was that if you eliminate fear and relax, having a baby is as simple as pie *only* if you're not neurotic. And of course we all are neurotic these days, so that lets us all out."

"Where did you say you read that?" asked her husband.

"I can't seem to remember," she said. "Now where was it?"

"That's a delightful theory," I began, "but it has nothing to do with the Pavlov method. The whole point of the Pavlov method is—"

"Please," said our new friend Ronnie, with a look of tight-lipped anguish, "is it absolutely necessary to discuss this while we eat?"

"What's the difference?" asked Shelley. "The chicken's spoiled anyway. Pass me your plate."

"Well what exactly *is* the Pavlov method then?" Gloria persisted. "It's all natural childbirth, isn't it? Don't misunderstand me, I think it's a fine idea. But it just doesn't work. My sister, Jinny, took a course in it, and she really tried. She and Hugo went all the way across town one evening a week for three whole months to study the thing. I don't think they *wasted* their time

—not entirely. But the fact is that when the time came, she was terribly disappointed. There *was* pain. And she wouldn't have minded a little pain, you understand. She really wanted to be there when the baby was born. She really did want to see it. . . ."

"Morbid curiosity," said Shelley.

"No. It would have meant a lot to her. Hugo knew he'd have to leave before the delivery, but she really thought she'd be there when the time came. Well, she wasn't. Her doctor told her afterward that he thought it was all a lot of nonsense. I suppose he was right. About the painless part, I mean. I can't see what he had against the education aspect. A little knowledge never hurt anyone."

"Oh, really," Ronnie said; "I don't see what you're all making such a fuss about. Listen, I have two children. Once they're in bed at night I put them out of my mind. Who cares how they get into the world? They're here! The whole project takes less than a day. What difference does it make if you're doped up or not? What difference does it make if you suffer a little? What difference does it make what the doctor believes in or says to you? You don't have to sleep with him. Everybody knows that doctors don't like natural childbirth. Everybody knows that they don't appreciate advice, and that they always do what they like no matter what they promise you. Who ever said that doctors are truthful—or even intelligent? You're getting a lot if they know their profession. Don't ask any more from them. They're only human after all— which is to say, you can't expect much."

"Take it easy, dear," her husband interrupted.

"That's just the point I'm trying to make! Take it easy! What is there to make a fuss about? Have a little perspective. What difference will any of it make in another hundred years?"

"What difference will anything make in another hundred years?" I tossed in.

After that no one mentioned childbirth for the rest of the evening. When we went home Alex and I made a pact never to discuss the subject in company again.

We didn't stick to it.

The reason for our failure to abstain was a telephone call from one of my childhood friends. I had seen her very infrequently since I had gone off to college, and I was surprised to hear from her again. "I had to talk to you," she began. "Your mother told me about the way you had Pepi and I thought you'd be interested to hear that I stumbled on something of the sort all by myself. I didn't like the way I had my first child, so I decided to wait as long as possible before going to the hospital for the second. By the time I got there, he was nearly born. I just sort of relaxed and panted and aside from a couple of difficult moments, I got through the whole thing without taking anything. It was a great thrill. More people ought to know about it."

"I'm glad you think so," I said, "but it's my impression that they don't want to know about it."

"No, really," she insisted, "if it's anything like what your mother described, it's tremendous. You ought to write an article about it. I'm sure a lot of people would be interested. I would."

"My God!" I said. "How many do you plan to have?"

"Oh, five or six. I've got another on the way right now. So you'd better hurry."

I repeated the conversation to Alex.

"Why don't you?" he asked.

"Six children!" That seemed like rather a handful.

"No," he said, "the article. People who are offended by the subject won't read it, and the ones who are interested in it will profit. And you'll have got it off your chest."

I wrote the article. I started from the very beginning and told the whole story right through to the end. I sent it off to a woman's magazine with the hope that it would make it easier for other women to arrive at my great adventure a little more directly than I had myself.

Several weeks later I received a telephone call from one of the editors of the magazine. He apologized for holding the article for so long. Did I mind his keeping it a little longer?

"Not at all," I said. "Why?"

"It's fascinating," was his answer. "But it's very controversial. There are several more people I want to read it."

Two months and several telephone conversations later the article was returned to me with a note to the effect that after lengthy discussion it had been vetoed as being too controversial. I was advised to keep sending it out, because someone would be sure to print it eventually. I privately chalked it up as a lost cause and not without regret. Only one thing puzzled me. "Controversial in what way?" I asked Alex. "The Russian part or the childbirth part?"

"Who knows," he answered. "Probably a little of both."

Then one day a girl I had met in Paris stopped around to chat with us on her way home to Detroit. She and her husband were discussing the problem of finding an apartment because she was going to have a baby. One thing led to another, and there we were again on the proscribed subject. No sooner had I got the word Pavlov out of my mouth than she became terribly excited.

"That's it!" she said. "That's the thing that was all over the French newspapers."

"That's right," we agreed.

"I want it!" she said. "That's the way I want to have my baby."

"Unfortunately I don't think it's possible," I said.

"Why on earth not?"

We tried to explain.

"It must be possible," she insisted. "Aren't there any books on the subject?"

I looked at Alex. We had a book on the subject. Colette Jeanson's book was sitting right there on the bookshelf. But how far could she go with only a book as a guide? Who could say? We all talked about what I had done in some detail and finally she took the book away with her, promising to let us know the outcome. I was very skeptical about her chances for success. I knew I shouldn't have liked to do it all alone. I was secure in the thought that I was going to return to Paris when I was ready to have another baby. Still, I admired her courage.

Then the day came when I announced to Alex that either Marianne or Philip (we have them all named way in advance) was probably on the way. The same thought occurred to us both simultaneously—it was impossible for us to go to France. For the first time we realized that parenthood had considerably decreased our mobility. I would have to have the baby in New York.

"Well why not?" Alex asked. "This is a very modern city. You've done it before. Just find a good young doctor, not too set in his ways, explain it all to him, and let me be your monitor. What could be easier?"

It sounded like the simplest thing in the world.

That afternoon I found myself magnetically drawn to the shelf on maternity at the corner bookshop. I got everything I could find on the subject. I wanted to know all about what to expect in an American maternity hospital. In one of the first books I picked up I came across this helpful bit of advice: "Shop around until you find a doctor you like." It struck me as a novel idea, and a useful one. But it is only now, after I've been through the whole thing, that I realize how important that advice really was. And how many pitfalls there are to avoid. That is why I devote the next few pages to the rather amusing experiences that eventually led me to the right man. *Caveat emptor!*

I began in my usual manner—with the telephone. I called a friend who moves largely in medical circles.

"Hello Cynthia," I said. "Do you happen to know where I can find a good obstetrician?"

"Congratulations," she said. "Just a minute. I'll get my little black book."

A short wait filled by the sounds of children breaking something at the other end of the line.

"Here you are. Got a pencil?"

I took down the name and number.

Then I called the doctor she recommended and made an appointment. I was in a hurry to get the whole matter settled.

When the day came, Alex came along with me. We had decided that he had better be present at the first visit, just in case the doctor should have any doubts about what I told him. Alex could serve as an unbiased eyewitness. As it turned out, the doctor didn't seem skeptical at all. He was an elderly and distinguished gentleman who inspired confidence. When I had finished telling my story, he leaned forward in his chair, and looked at us both intently for a minute. Then he said: "You are unusual people."

"In any particular way?" I asked, not sure what was coming next.

He leaned back again and lit his pipe. He began to relate how he had always delivered without any drugs thirty or so years before. In his opinion it was much easier on everyone concerned. Then, he said, when heavy anesthesia became the fashion, he had had to use it, like everyone else. For a while it was a dangerous affair, especially for the infant. But of course everyone had to have it. Now, however, it was vastly improved, and he felt better about the whole question. "But," he said, "it's a rare pleasure to meet people who don't coddle themselves."

"But there are lots of women who have children without anesthesia these days," I protested.

"No," he shook his head, "no, there aren't. The women don't want it. And after all you must give people what they want. This is a profession like any other."

I was not too certain about the logic or the morality of that statement. Still, I hadn't come to pass judgment on his character. For the next half hour he detailed for us his student exploits on the Left Bank in 1910. It was all settled when we arose to leave.

Alex was to be present at the delivery, which would be performed without any drugs of any kind—unless I were to change my mind at the time, in which case he would certainly oblige. I assured him that, barring any emergency, there would be no change of plan.

"Yes indeed," he said, getting up to show us to the door, "I am glad that you feel the way you do. You are very courageous people. I'm for it. That's the way we were in my day. We believed in letting nature take its course. No pampering. No fuss about the facts of life. Women knew they had to suffer to bring forth and that was that. You shall bring forth in pain. No one tried to dodge the issue. Childbirth *is* painful. Now we know how to alleviate suffering somewhat. But is it really worth it? And doesn't it show that we have weakened in our moral fiber? And how about all the youth crimes today?"

"What about them?" I asked, totally lost.

"Out of a woman's suffering springs her mother love," he declaimed rhetorically. "I don't say you can prove it, but I fervently believe in the connection." He looked to Alex significantly, as though that were the sort of thing only another man could be expected to appreciate.

"But that isn't the Pavlov method at all," I began. I caught Alex's eye and shut up. What was the use?

"Of course," the doctor sighed philosophically, "if a woman wants to be pampered then we are forced to pamper her. But it's a pleasure to meet someone who doesn't. My secretary will make you an appointment."

We shook hands seriously and said good-bye. We slipped past the secretary who was talking on the phone, and started to laugh as soon as we hit the open air.

"And I thought we had a real understanding," I said.

The next day I telephoned to say that we had suddenly been called out of town. It wasn't worth the effort to try to explain my way through his philosophical convictions of forty years' standing.

We decided that the easiest way would be to find someone who already practiced his own system of "natural" childbirth, and to try to persuade him to cooperate with us on ours.

I asked around again and finally turned up a genial-sounding name at a very reliable address on Park Avenue. I was assured that this man was "very much up on the latest in natural childbirth." Just to be certain, when I called for an appointment, I asked the receptionist if she felt the doctor could be talked into trying a new method of natural childbirth. The question appeared to offend her deeply. "Everyone knows," she reproved me, "that he always tries to give his patients exactly what they want so long as it is in keeping with sound medical practice." I felt as though I had just asked for an illegal supply of drugs.

Still, I refused to be put off by a receptionist, so I made an appointment for the following Tuesday. By this time I thought I knew what to look for, and I told Alex he wouldn't have to waste any more time on these sorties. I could finish the shopping alone.

After waiting the ritual hour I was singled out by the receptionist to begin work on my dossier. When the question period was over, a very starchy nurse came to escort me to the changing room and afterwards into a small examining parlor where I was weighed and measured and then told to "hop up on the table like a good girl." I imagined that the aim of this treatment was to have the patient properly humble and subdued before she even met the doctor. "I would prefer to talk things over sitting up first, if you don't mind," I told the nurse.

"I'm sorry," she said. "We have a routine in this office. The doctor is a very busy man. You can't expect us to make exceptions for everyone." I looked down at the little white gown I was wearing, my stockings drooping down about my ankles, and realized how impossible it was to argue with her.

Suddenly the door opened, and into the room whisked a little sandy-haired fellow in his late fifties, graying and bespectacled.

He came around to the head of the table and peered intently into my face for a long minute.

"Well, well, well," he said. "What's the trouble here?"

"No trouble at all," I said, surprised out of my self-consciousness. "I'm lying here because of your routine, but what I really wanted was to talk to you about having a particular kind of delivery without any anesthetics. . . ."

"Certainly, certainly," he cut in in a pixyish tone, wrapping a long blood-pressure thing about my arm. "I'll give you anything you want."

"But I'd like to discuss it with you first. . . ."

"Shhh. Not now." He was pumping up the tube intently. "We can talk it all over later."

"No," I said. "Now. Because if you don't want to do it, we won't have to go on with this. It's a system called the Pavlov method that was—"

"Just what is it that's so special it can't wait?" he said, pulling down my lower lid and peering at my eye. He shook his head and clucked sadly over what he saw there.

"For one thing, I want my husband to be there—*in the delivery room,* and then, *no* drugs of any kind, and then—"

"By all means," he interrupted, "what's so difficult about that?"

"Also, I'd like you to rehearse with us, so that we'll all be able to cooperate during the expulsion," I added.

"I told you, I'll do anything you want," he said with a note of impatience. I decided to drop the subject until some later time. After all, he had agreed to the two most important conditions.

He began his examination of my interior. There was a long silence. I lifted my head a little to see what accounted for it. His face was screwed up into the expression a watchmaker wears when he is engaged in the repair of a particularly tiny and difficult watch. At last he looked up with an air of measured consideration and authority: "You're not pregnant, Mrs. Karmel, you're sick."

If I hadn't been sick before, I was then. My stomach flipped over, and my heart began to pound wildly. Suddenly, before I had time to assemble my thoughts, he seized a little object from a tray, and came around and pierced my finger with it. He quickly blotted up a little drop of my blood on a piece of paper and held it under a color chart. "There!" he exclaimed showing it to me triumphantly. "Would you say it matched this or this?"

He slid my little blood spot back and forth between the red patch labeled thirty and the one marked forty. "Let's say thirty-five," he compromised. What was he doing? Was I to be integrated into his wife's living-room décor? He snatched up a little white card from the table and jotted on it "Hemoglobin thirty-five."

"It's a wonder you had the energy to get here at all," he said happily. "Fortunately that's something that's easy to fix." I sat stunned on the table while he bustled around preparing a large hypodermic. When he had finished the injection, he folded his arms and looked at me earnestly. "Has anyone ever told you, Mrs. Karmel, that you have a retroverted uterus?"

"Yes," I said, "often."

"Let me explain what is meant by that term," he began, and he embarked on a long and diagrammatic description that made my uterus sound rather like a balloon moored to my body by four over-long ligaments, without which it would drift up into outer space. "In any event," he concluded, "we can be certain that you will never be able to conceive a child until this condition has been remedied. Now I realize what a disappointment it is to you. But you are not pregnant, and unless we try to correct the situation it is not likely that you ever will be. I'm sure you had some reason to *think* yourself pregnant, but I want to try to get across to you that a woman may bring about many of the signs of pregnancy merely as the result of her intense longing for a child."

"Hand me my pocketbook," I said. I had put it on the window ledge. Looking perplexed, he gave it to me and I reached for my wallet. "There," I said holding out an especially cute picture of Pepi in a bathing suit. "I have not only conceived a child, but I have given birth to him. He did result from an intense longing, but he is not imaginary in the least."

The doctor proceeded to a re-examination of the problem. "Sure enough!" he exclaimed a few minutes later. "Now I can see that you're two months gone!"

I made a mental note of the word "gone." "How did you happen to make such a mistake?" I asked with malice.

"With a condition like yours," he answered, "it is often difficult to be certain at such an early stage. Now that you are pregnant," he went on, giving the impression that in some way he considered himself responsible for my sudden success, "I want you to leave everything to me. When your time comes, I will do everything in my power to make things easy for you. And I'll try to be with you as much as possible."

"You won't have to do that," I said. "That's my husband's job."

"Your husband?"

"He's going to be there with me," I reminded him.

"Oh, certainly, he can be there. Yes, I'll arrange to have him stay with you right up until we put you out."

"No," I corrected him. "You aren't going to put me out. You agreed that I wasn't going to have any anesthesia. . . ."

"Of course, of course," he said, "no one's going to do anything you don't want them to. We can arrange all the details later. Your husband can certainly stay with you in the labor room if that's what you want."

"And the delivery room."

"And the deliv— Why? What's he going to do in the delivery room? Is he studying medicine? Why does he have to go to the delivery room?"

"Because I want him there. In the Pavlov method—"

"What difference does it make to you? Once we put you out—"

"I'm not going out, remember?"

"Oh yes, of course. Well, perhaps we can arrange to have the delivery in the labor room, if you really think you're not going to need anything."

"We can arrange the details some other time," I said.

The minute I got home I called to cancel my next appointment. I gave the reason as a "change of mind."

Then I telephoned Cynthia again for another name. From my first two experiences I had deduced that hers was the more reliable source. I explained that I was still shopping. "Come on over and have a drink," she said, "and tell me what you've found."

I did. She made a potent martini, and I told my tale. When she had finished laughing, she assured me that that wasn't the sort of thing that happened to one twice. "You'll never stumble on another one like that," she said, "not in a million years. Most doctors are perfectly sane."

"I can forgive insanity," I said, "but not lying. How can a doctor say he's going to do one thing when he really intends to do another?"

"That part's easy enough to understand," she said.

"It is? Why?"

"Good God," she said. "If you ever saw the women who come into an obstetrician's office in a single day, you'd even wonder why they all haven't gone mad. They couldn't be entirely truthful and survive it." Then she told me a few stories to illustrate the stupidity of women.

"That's all very interesting," I said. "But how do you excuse a doctor's saying he practices childbirth without anesthesia when he doesn't? After all, that question has nothing to do with anyone's intelligence. It ought to be perfectly simple to answer it truthfully. Either he practices it or he doesn't."

"Not that easy," she said, pouring another round.

"Why isn't it?"

"In the first place, lots of women say they want 'natural' childbirth without any idea of what they mean. They don't really want it at all."

"And how does a doctor determine that?"

"From past experience. When it first came out lots of young doctors thought it was a great idea. They recommended books and courses to take. They were really ready to go along with it. But when things got rough, practically every woman shouted for help. Now they think it's just a joke. So they've worked it out to everyone's satisfaction. If a woman wants 'natural' childbirth, they give it to her. They tell her where to get the information and the exercises. They say they practice it. When the time comes they go ahead and put the woman out. When she wakes up, she says 'Isn't it marvelous? I had my baby by natural childbirth.' She's pleased with herself and the doctor has a good laugh. Everybody's happy. What's wrong with that?"

"But it's lying!" I said. "That's what's wrong with it."

"Suppose it is? It's dealing with the problem in a realistic manner. The woman is always perfectly happy; she thinks she's had natural childbirth, whatever that is."

"I see. You think it's perfectly reasonable and moral for a doctor to have his own standards of truth and falsehood?"

She smiled thoughtfully and tapped out a cigarette from the pack on the table. She looked at it reflectively. "Yes, I do. I think it should be up to his own discretion to modify the truth as he sees fit. If you ever worked for a doctor, you'd know how difficult it would be for him if he were always forced to stick to the literal truth."

"Morality is difficult for everybody."

"Oh go on! Have another drink!"

"Then the fact is almost every doctor I approach about the Pavlov method is going to pretend to agree to do it?"

"I shouldn't be surprised."

"But without really meaning it at all?"

"That's very possible. But of course, it will be up to you to find that out."

"Great!" I said. "That's just peachy. I think I'll try to get to Paris after all."

I was ready to drop the whole question right there! I would find any competent man to go to for my monthly check-ups, and when the time came I would go to Paris. With a little fancy arithmetic I even persuaded myself that, plane fare included, the whole trip probably wouldn't amount to more than the cost of having the baby in New York City. When another friend recommended that I see a doctor she knew, I agreed to use him as the temporary stop-gap. "Do you think he'll mind my just seeing him for check-ups?" I asked her. "I'll just tell him I have to go abroad the month before the delivery. I won't even bother to mention the Pavlov method."

"Oh no," she protested, "you ought to tell him about it. Who knows, he might be just the man you're looking for? I'm sure he'll go along with it, if anybody will. Really, he's terribly modern and advanced. He has an open mind. You ought to give him a chance."

Naturally I agreed to see him.

He turned out to be very young. He hid this fact, as best he could, behind a thick layer of complacent-looking fat. He had a habit of staring earnestly into your face without blinking for long stretches of time. No doubt that accounted for his bloodshot eyes, although it is possible that the dim light of his office might alone be responsible. I could not tell whether he was suffering from a bad cold, or whether it was merely the impact of the atmosphere that made him whisper. Whatever the cause, the malady was contagious. I was well advanced in what seemed to me about the fiftieth recounting of my saga, when I realized that I was whispering too.

He stared at me intently as I tried to explain the essence of the Pavlov method. When I finished I paused and waited for him to ask any questions that he might have. He stared at me intently. We both waited.

"Well," I said finally. "Is there anything that seems unclear?"

"Yes," he said after a brief silence. "Now, Marjorie—how did you become involved with this . . . affair?"

"Oh," I laughed, "that's a long story." He said nothing. A minute passed very slowly. I assumed that he was waiting to hear the story. And so I began. Fortunately he redirected his penetrating gaze to a corner of the ceiling while I spoke.

Suddenly he broke in, his eyes still fixed on the distant corner. "Marjorie, you say you had made two hospital reservations? One in Paris and one in New York?"

"Yes," I said.

"Wouldn't you say that it was a little over-cautious of you?" he asked. "And you saw two doctors. Do you think the average person would have been so fastidious about the preliminary examinations in the unsettled circumstances you described to me?"

"I don't know anything about averages," I answered, beginning to be annoyed. "I know that a pregnant woman should see a doctor once a month and a dentist twice a year. I try to do as I'm told. Better cautious than careless, isn't that what they always say?"

He smiled disarmingly. "I don't mean to antagonize you, Marjorie," he said. "But I want to understand you very thoroughly. I believe that a physician's duty goes beyond the simple practice of his skill. He must understand his patient in every sense. He must be a friend, a confidant. The patient must feel free to express all her worries, her anxieties. You seem to be an educated person, Marjorie. You must know something about psychology. Then you will understand what I mean when I say that in obstetrics as in psychoanalysis, for the doctor-patient relationship to have a valid meaning, there must be a transference, the doctor must be a sort of father image."

I sat back, stunned. I tried to imagine why there ought to be a transference, or why the relationship between doctor and patient needed any valid meaning beyond the obvious one of honesty and skill on the part of the physician, and cooperation and the ability to pay the fee on the part of the patient. "Really," I protested, "I don't want a father image. I just want to have my baby by the Pavlov method."

"You can't expect me to help you unless I know the entire story," he said. "You must try to be completely honest with me, Marjorie."

"I have been."

There was no answer. He had fixed another spot on the ceiling, and was leaning back in his chair again, expectantly stroking his chin. I assumed that was my cue to go on with my story. I shortened it as much as I could, hoping to end the interview as soon as possible.

Again he interrupted. "Would you mind going back just a bit and repeating what you just said?"

"Which?" I had said a great deal.

"The part about Mme. Cohen's eyes when she appeared in the doorway. Would you repeat your description of her eyes?"

I saw what was coming. "I said she had large eyes," I said slowly, "large, bright, beautiful eyes. It was a pleasure to see her, and I was *not* hypnotized."

He smiled smugly.

"Look, Doctor," I said getting up, "I appreciate your technique, but I honestly don't believe that we are going to be compatible."

"You must believe in my sincerity, Marjorie," he said, "when I say that I can assure you a more meaningful experience here than the one you had in France. I think you will find that my methods are *very* sympathetic to your temperament. If you like, I'll try to arrange to have music for you during your labor."

"Whatever for?"

"I have a friend who is a dentist who has had extraordinary results with it in the dental chair. Actually, I welcome the opportunity to try it out."

"No, thank you," I said. "It would ruin my concentration." I hadn't gone there to discuss the healing powers of music. I got up to leave.

"Think over all we've said, Marjorie," he said, taking my hand and sandwiching it between his. "Then let me know if we are going to go ahead. I don't want to force you into a decision. You must find your own way . . ."

"I will," I said.

That evening, when I had told the whole story to Alex, something suddenly occurred to me. "I know it sounds silly," I said, "but for some reason what annoyed me as much as anything else was his calling me by my first name. Why should that be?"

"I hope you called him by his first name too," Alex said.

"Of course not," I answered.

"Well next time make sure you do," he ordered.

"But Alex, he's a *doctor*. I couldn't!"

"Then that explains why you were annoyed," Alex said. "One-way first-name calling always means inequality—witness servants, children, and dogs."

"Dr. Lamaze always called me madame," I said. "I don't see that our relation was any the worse for it. As a matter of fact, Mme. Cohen always called me Mme. Karmel. And it never would have occurred to me to call her Blanche. I think that just made it easier to be frank about intimate details."

"Darling," Alex said, "this is America. When in Rome . . ."

The point was well taken. I decided to forget the whole matter for at least three weeks. My feet hurt.

Then Cynthia called again. "My spouse just read an article in the paper," she said. "It seems that just yesterday a panel discussion was held at some local medical school on the subject of the Pavlov method. There was a hot dispute—or a warm chat at any rate. What do you think of that?"

"Bravo!" I said. "Someone has heard of it at last."

"Think some more."

"I suppose that if there was a dispute, or even a warm chat, then someone must have been in favor of the Pavlov method. The problem now is to discover who."

"Get your pencil out," she said. And that was how I came to find Dr. Sedley.

I was not terribly hopeful when I walked into his office. I didn't want to be disappointed again. His appearance was encouraging. He *looked* like a sensible man. He was young and good-looking, and, say what you will, that is always a help.

I rattled out my story as fast as I could. I was in a hurry to find out whether or not he could really do the Pavlov method. All I asked, I said, was to be permitted to have no anesthesia unless I asked for it, to be permitted to deal with my own labor in my own way, and above all, that Alex be present the whole time, including the delivery itself. When I had finished, he thought for a moment and said "What you have just described sounds more like the Read method than like what I know of the Pavlov method."

"It isn't like the Read method," I said, a little taken aback.

"It sounds much more humane than the Pavlov method," he said. "Except for the part where Mme. Cohen throws cold water in your face. I would never permit that sort of brutality."

"Oh, that wasn't brutal," I explained. "It was wonderful. It was just what I needed."

"I've read about how they use the Pavlov method in Russia," he said, "but I've only actually seen it in Italy. There it impressed me as being too crude for any American woman to stand for—or be expected to stand for—a great number of women all herded together in one room with a lot of relatives and noise, having their babies together to music."

"I can't believe that had anything to do with the Pavlov method," I said. "But that's not the point. What I want is to have my baby the way I did in Paris—whatever you want to call it. It was wonderful, and I'd like to have the same thing again."

"Well, I'll do everything *I* can to help you," he said reassuringly. "As a matter of fact, I think we can work out something even better than what you had in Paris. I'll try to find a nurse to be your *monitrice*. Not only will your husband be there, but I'll be there with you the entire time myself. No one will give you any drugs unless you ask for them. I think you'll like the hospital very much. I can't say that I believe in the Pavlov method, but I'm willing to have you show me and I'll do everything I can to help."

It was such delightful news that I almost burst into tears. Surely I couldn't have asked for anything more. "Thank you, Dr. Sedley," I said. "That's a tremendous relief!"

"And Marjorie," he added, "please don't hesitate to call on me if you need me at any time. I hope you will think of me as a friend. I believe in the importance of the relationship between the doctor and his patient."

There it was again! The first name combined with the psychological relationship. Well, I thought, I can take it. In France there had been the insistent "*C'est belle, n'est-ce pas?*" In America there seemed to be psychology. I supposed I could learn to live with that. It was certainly worth the effort.

We discussed some of the details of what I wanted, and Dr. Sedley promised to arrange things at the hospital as best he could. Then he examined me, and pronounced me in fine shape. I went away convinced that at last I had found a doctor who was honest, kind and intelligent. We weren't in total agreement about the Pavlov method, but at least he had heard of it. I hoped that I would be able to demonstrate how good it was. But what was most important was that he was willing to let me try.

I rushed home to tell Alex the good news. I was halfway through the recital when the phone rang. Alex answered it. "For you," he said. "Some doctor. I didn't catch the name."

I took the receiver. It was doctor number two. "I see you canceled your appointment," he said. "Would you mind telling me why?"

"Not at all," I answered, surprised at who it was. "If you remember, I was looking for someone to deliver my baby without anesthesia and with my husband present in the delivery room. By the end of my visit I could see that you weren't going to go along with that."

"I don't mean to go poking my nose in unwanted," he said, "but what makes you think you're going to find any respectable doctor who will?"

"I've already found one," I said. "It's all settled."

"It isn't really my business," the doctor said, "but I'm driven to say this to you out of a sense of duty. I can't imagine what kind of a quack you've got mixed up with, but I can tell you that no self-respecting physician is going to let your husband step one foot into that delivery room!"

"But I'm afraid this one is, Doctor. It's all settled."

"What's the fellow's name?"

"I'm sorry, but I don't—"

"Well, that's all right, but you had better believe me, you're going to regret the whole thing."

"I don't think so, Doctor. I've done it before, you know."

Alex was making questioning gestures from across the room. The conversation must have sounded wild on just one end. I was tempted to prolong it just to tease him.

"Yes," the doctor said. "That's all very well if everything goes along all right. A normal delivery is nothing . . . but what's that doctor going to do when something goes wrong? What's he going to do with a hysterical husband pushing his elbow around? Yes sir, when the birth is normal it's like pulling a cork out of the bottle, but what's that fellow going to do when he has to go in with the corkscrew? You just tell me that!"

"I don't know, Doctor," I answered, putting the receiver gently back on its cradle. "Just wait till I tell you this one, darling," I said, somewhat hysterical. "You'll never believe it."

8 *The Birds and the Bees*

I've described what it was like finding a doctor who would let me do the Pavlov method in an American hospital because I think any woman might run into the same thing. In this chapter I'm going to describe what it was like to take a course in "natural childbirth" at an American hospital, because any woman who wants to do the Pavlov method in America is likely to run into something very much like it, and she ought to be warned of the pitfalls before she begins. I'd be much happier if there were some place all set up to teach the Pavlov method as it should be taught, and all I had to do was tell how good it was. But for the present there isn't, and anyone who feels as I do that the Pavlov method with its direct and frank attack on the causes of pain in childbirth is superior to other varieties of childbirth without anesthesia is going to find herself out of step in even the best American institution. And she had better be-prepared for it.

My decision to take the course at the hospital was not prompted by intellectual curiosity. Dr. Sedley had promised to arrange everything, and I had a conviction that he would keep his word. It wasn't until my second visit that I began to realize that you could not just walk into a hospital and do what you liked. A hospital, after all, is an institution, which is to say a little like Kafka's *The Castle.*

"Well, Marjorie, I've done my best to arrange things," Dr. Sedley greeted me. "If all goes well, your husband will be allowed in the delivery room."

"If all goes well?"

"It's only fair to warn you that some of the rooms are too small to hold an extra person. But if the floor isn't crowded, we'll have a big room and I'll see that he's there."

"But really," I protested. "Nothing could be smaller than the delivery room at the Belvédère, and it held everybody very nicely. Alex doesn't take up all that room."

"It's a matter of hospital policy," he replied. "Another problem is the *monitrice*. I'm fairly sure I can find someone to practice with you, but I can't promise that she'll be with you during the delivery. The nurses all have fixed schedules."

I thought that one over for a minute. "What good will that do me?" I asked finally.

"She can help you with your exercises."

"But I know the exercises already. What I need is guidance during the delivery."

"That's true. Perhaps I can find a student nurse who'd be willing to try it."

"Actually I think I can do perfectly well without a *monitrice*. Alex knows all about it."

"I don't think you need to worry," he assured me. "I'll be with you, and the nurses are very good. They have a lot of experience with natural childbirth; as a matter of fact they give an excellent course right at the hospital. As long as you're willing to meet them halfway, I'm sure things will work out all right."

The prospect of meeting something new halfway in the middle of labor was not altogether delightful. At school I had learned that it was never wise to break the rules until I knew them. Hospitals were probably the same. "Perhaps I'll take that course in natural childbirth," I suggested. "Then I'll know what to expect."

"That might not be a bad idea."

I arrived at the hospital on the appointed day and hour prepared to sit in the back row of the classroom and take notes. I very quickly realized that I should have left my notebook at home. It was not going to be a lecture course, but a discussion group. There were only eight women in the class and together with Miss Smiley, the teacher, we sat in a cozy little circle at one end of a large airy room. This circular arrangement might have created the intimate social atmosphere that was intended had it not been for the row of mats that stretched out behind us on the floor. Probably if we had got directly down on the mats and done any exercise whatsoever, we should all have felt at ease within five minutes. But as it happened they lay there behind us for nearly two full sessions (four hours), empty and mildly threatening, while we delicately discussed the problem of what to wear when we finally did get down on them. Meanwhile the circular arrangement gave us an excellent view of each other's silhouettes, which varied wildly.

Miss Smiley began by asking us to introduce ourselves. We turned out to be a wide assortment of individuals, each with different past experiences and different expectations from the course. Miss Smiley's method of teaching soon became clear. She wasn't going to tell us; we were going to tell her. For eight two-hour sessions we were going to discuss all the questions we had on our minds, take a tour of the hospital, then have a night session with our husbands to deal with their questions. At the proper moment Miss Smiley would show us a few simple, helpful exercises. She was only there to help us; it was *our* class.

We began by discussing the term "natural childbirth." We considered what we thought it meant, what other people thought it meant, whether it existed at all, whether it was primitive, barbaric, hypnotic, stoic, modern, or old-fashioned. We tried to decide whether natural meant painless, and whether childbirth really could be painless. We got a little heated on that point. I said it could be. But a very pretty young lady who had had two children with caudal anesthesia (which she swore was the most advanced and best) claimed that I was lying, and that childbirth meant pain. A girl who had had one child by the Read method said it could be nearly painless. Miss Smiley calmed the discussion with the comment that everyone reacts differently. We discussed all kinds of pains. Miss Smiley assured us that whenever we wanted it anesthesia would be available.

If I had realized the effect all this was having on me, I would have left immediately. But I had forgotten about the possibility of becoming deconditioned. By the end of the first class I had begun to wonder what would happen to me if I did lose control without Mme. Cohen there to help me back.

We went through two sessions of this. I began to wonder why Miss Smiley never spoke up. I watched her conduct the class, sweetly, deferentially, listening to what everyone said, nodding approvingly from time to time. You are all individuals, she seemed to say. I respect your right to believe whatever you choose. I am not here to demand anything of you. I am not here to shock you. I am not going to sell you anything. But at the same time I wondered what I would have felt if I had come to this class after I had decided that childbirth without anesthesia was the thing for me but still knew very little about it. Mightn't it have been like being not able to find a salesgirl when you want to buy?

"How do you feel about getting down on the mats today?" Miss Smiley asked the next time we met.

"Enthusiastic," I answered. I did not look forward to more discussion.

We sat tailor fashion in our slips. Then we talked some more. In the course of the conversation we managed to slip in a few posture and limbering exercises. Then we turned to relaxation. Miss Smiley brought out a lot of pillows and we experimented with various positions to find which was the most comfortable. The idea was to think of music or waves at the seashore or any-thing else that was soothing. We shut our eyes and Miss Smiley tiptoed about testing an ankle here and a wrist there to see that they were relaxed. I found it quite pleasurable to lie stretched out on my little mat in the dim light (Miss Smiley had pulled down the shades). It reminded me of nap time in the kindergarten I had attended. We had all relaxed and imagined the Sandman was putting us to sleep while the shadow of the leaves outside flickered softly over the floor. The contrast with Mme. Cohen's exercise in muscular control could not have been more complete.

The next session we took up abdominal breathing. It so happens that I have been taught abdominal breathing at frequent intervals during my life. I have been thoroughly impressed with its importance for sports, acting, singing, speaking, and general well-being. The curious thing is I don't believe I've ever used it for anything outside of a class. Naturally I was interested to see it applied to childbirth.

We lay on our backs with one hand on the rib cage and the other on the abdomen. The idea was to take a slow, deep breath that would not expand the ribs at all, but push straight down on the diaphragm, making the abdomen rise. That much was easy. Miss Smiley explained that we should practice taking as long as possible about it so that we could begin to inhale at the start of the contraction and not exhale until the contraction had passed its peak. The point was that the abdominal wall would be lifted away from the uterus by the breathing, and that to let it fall back again too soon might disturb the uterus at its work. I wondered what effect the diaphragm might be having on the uterus in the meantime. But as no one else brought up the question, I let it pass.

"How long is a contraction?" someone asked.

Miss Smiley explained that early contractions might be about thirty seconds long. She timed us with her stop watch and was proud that we all made the grade.

"But as labor goes on," she said, "they get longer and longer."

"How long?"

"Oh, a minute or even more."

We tried it. Obviously no one could do it.

"When you can't keep inhaling right up to the peak, there is something else you can do," Miss Smiley explained. "Inhale as long as you can. Then take a series of little panting breaths, not in the chest, but in the same abdominal way so that the abdomen does not sink down, but just flutters a little. When the peak is past, exhale slowly all the way. Here, let me show you."

Lying flat on her back, she began to inhale. Her stomach puffed up higher and higher for about twenty seconds, then it rose and fell very slightly for another twenty seconds, then at last it slowly sank back to its customary flatness. It was an extraordinary performance.

We tried it. The results were ludicrous.

"Don't worry if you can't do it right away," Miss Smiley said. "Remember that I've had years of practice."

No matter what frame of mind I had come to the course with, I think my confidence would have been shaken at that point if I was counting on abdominal breathing to get me through labor. What pregnant woman had years to spend in practice? Someone else had the same thought. "What happens if we haven't learned to do that when the time comes?" she asked.

"Well you can always take another breath," Miss Smiley said. "Just do the best you can and relax. Remember it's not a contest. The nurse will probably give you a little Demerol if you have any trouble relaxing. Remember there will always be nurses in and out, ready to help you."

After class I couldn't restrain myself any more. "Miss Smiley," I said, "in France they taught me a much easier way to deal with contractions. If you just breathe with your *chest*, the uterus and abdomen are left perfectly undisturbed. And it's so much easier to learn."

"That's very interesting," she said. "A Belgian doctor visited us a couple of years ago and said they weren't using abdominal breathing over there any more. But, unfortunately, he was only here for a day. He never told us what they use instead."

"Chest breathing," I said. "And panting when that isn't sufficient."

"We use panting during the expulsion."

"It works marvelously before."

She nodded thoughtfully, but that was all we ever said about the subject.

"How do you all feel about looking at pictures?" she asked when we arrived the next time.

I thought how delicate her approach was compared to Mme. Cohen's. We all looked at each other as though the answer lay somewhere in the collective subconscious. No one wanted to look overly eager. Suddenly the girl who had had the Read method launched into an enthusiastic account of a movie she had seen of a delivery. Someone else said she wouldn't mind looking at pictures if they weren't too bad. Eventually everyone agreed that they might look at some pictures. "What do you think?" Miss Smiley asked me.

"Well," I said, "I think the knowledge and assurance they give you is well worth the initial shock."

"Since we're all agreed that it's a good idea, maybe we will look at some pictures next time."

All through the next class, which was another kaffeeklatsch, I wondered when we were going to look at the pictures. But nothing more was said about them, and I concluded they must be pretty gruesome. At last, just as we were about to leave, Miss Smiley asked again, "What would you say to looking at some pictures next week?"

This time I kept out of the discussion. Obviously there was something horrifying about those pictures. If Miss Smiley was so reluctant to show them, probably it wasn't a good idea to see them at all. Mme. Cohen's pictures had been upsetting enough before

I came to terms with myself, but these must be worse. And then I felt a sudden disgust for myself and all humanity as well. How had we managed to get into a state where the sight of a healthy woman giving birth to a healthy child could be so strange and upsetting?

The next week, Miss Smiley kept her word. She appeared with a stack of huge cardboard plates. So that's it, I said to myself. Cinemascope. Her hesitation now seemed perfectly understandable to me—I find the sight of two people's oversized faces in a close-up embrace pretty revolting whenever I go to the movies. I was ready to squirm. Miss Smiley turned over the first picture. It was a full-sized reproduction of one of those frequently published plates from the Maternity Center. It was a picture all right, but it was a picture of a plaster model of a cross section of a woman's abdomen showing the infant *in utero*. It was unimaginable that it could be disturbing to anyone. In fact, the implication was insulting. As for that thrilling and breath-taking sight, the entrance of a live baby into the world, we were left to guess what it might look like. If I hadn't known already, by now I would certainly have imagined it to be a spectacle of unparalleled gore.

I don't mean to say that the pictures of the plaster models weren't excellent. They were the same ones Mme. Cohen had shown me in Paris. The lecture that went with them was full and interesting, teaching in the simplest sense of the word. At last Miss Smiley admitted that she knew more than we did. Plate by plate she showed us the child's progress from the uterus down the birth canal. She pointed out just what was happening at every stage, what muscles were at work in the uterus, what they were accomplishing, what was happening to the sack of waters and the baby's head, how long it would take, and what sensations the mother might experience. When she described the delivery of the head she used a doll just as Mme. Cohen had. She assured us that the baby's head could get through without causing harm. (But *seeing*, as they say, is believing.) Her references to what the woman was to do while all this was going on were rather limited. The mother could breathe abdominally or chest-breathe a little, relax, and finally, expel the baby by taking a big breath, holding it, and pushing the way you push for a bowel movement. "Suddenly you're going to feel as though you had a grapefruit in your rectum," she explained. "Obviously you'll want to get it out as fast as possible." She demonstrated this, gulping and grimacing, growing redder and redder in the face. Then she let out her breath, shook her head, and laughed. "There you are! Contraction over."

She performed this little exhibition while we were all sitting tailor fashion on the floor. It did not really convey any idea of what it would be like to push while lying flat on your back on the delivery table. I remembered Mme. Cohen's warning about the dangers of associating pushing during the expulsion with emptying the bowels. But fortunately Miss Smiley obviated some of this danger by teaching us an exercise for relaxing the pelvic floor.

And that was all we were to learn about the delivery itself. It was all good—as far as it went. If I had had my first child knowing only that much I would certainly have been relieved of the anxiety of having something completely unknown happen to me. On the other hand, I would have been left completely passive and dependent. There was no real step-by-step training in how to conduct your own labor. There was nothing like the feeling of confidence I got from Mme. Cohen's insistence that *I* would be the one who would have my baby.

The sight of the plates reawakened the old discussion of the possibility of painless childbirth. The caudal girl glared at me suddenly from the next mat.

"Don't say it!" she warned. "Don't try to tell me childbirth isn't painful! If you try to tell me that it isn't, I'll just hate you!"

"Of course it's painful," I said. "But it doesn't *have* to be. You

can *learn* to do something about it. Just because an untrained
child will drown if you throw him in the water doesn't mean that
it is impossible to learn to swim."

"Nevertheless!" she said. Obviously, caudal or no, she had suffered badly in her first two deliveries. She refused to admit that
her suffering might have been in vain. She repeated how much
she liked caudals and how she hoped to be able to have one again.
Miss Smiley calmed the discussion with the customary hymn to
the highly differentiated individual.

We went on to talk about various kinds of anesthesia. We ana-
lyzed twilight sleep. It was generally felt that if the only effect of
scopolamine was to make you forget your suffering when it was
over, it might just as well be left out of the cocktail. Trilene,
someone said, smelled bad and worked notoriously too little and
too late. Spinals and caudals might be dangerous unless adminis-
tered just right. The hero of the day turned out to be Demerol.

"But what does Demerol do?" someone asked.

"It helps you relax. It takes the edge off pain."

"I see. What's it like?"

"Supposing you took two or three martinis. You'd be pretty relaxed, wouldn't you?"

"I'd be out cold," I said. "And in no condition to concentrate
on having a baby."

"Could I have the martinis instead?" someone asked.

Demerol, it was decided, would probably suffice until you
moved into the delivery room for the expulsion. Then a fascinating
assortment of gases and local anesthetics would be available to
supplement it. I found this astonishing. I have not yet met anyone
who went into the expulsion stage in full control who did not find
it the least difficult part of the delivery. In fact it is usually
described as a moment of intense joy. The idea of cheating yourself
of that reward for all the hard work of labor by taking gas seemed
senseless to me. Yet somehow it seems to be done more often
than not.

I found all this discussion of anesthesia discouraging. But obviously it was only intended to be reassuring. "You must not think of it as a contest," Miss Smiley repeated again and again. "If you need drugs don't feel ashamed to take them. Every one of you is an individual."

I couldn't help contrasting this speech with Mme. Cohen's repeated pep talks. Mme. Cohen insisted it *was* a sporting event. Her reassurance consisted of reminding me that she and Dr. Lamaze and the nurses would all be on my team backing me up. Certainly Miss Smiley was right when she said that no one should feel ashamed of taking drugs when she needed them. But it seems to me to be bad coaching to send you out on the field already resigned to defeat. I do think of labor as a contest. And I think it is worth taking the trouble to win.

On each of my visits to Dr. Sedley he asked me what I thought of the course at the hospital. Until it was over, I said only that I couldn't pass judgment because I hadn't yet seen all of it. The third time he asked I had to admit that I felt it left a lot to be desired.

"It's excellent general education that ought to be given in every high school," I said. "But I don't think it really prepares you to take an active part in the birth of your child."

"It isn't taught in every high school," Dr. Sedley pointed out. "Girls come to me who have no idea what's going to happen to them. Some of them are scared to death. That course gives them a real sense of knowledge, a real peace of mind. They aren't all like you; many of them don't have the self-confidence to take kindly to the suggestion that having their babies is their responsibility. It wouldn't be fair to foist a single point of view on them. The object is to help everyone."

"And to offend no one?"

"You have to consider the women you're dealing with. Many of them don't want . . ."

"And many of them do. What about them?" I asked. "Don't you think they should be given a little consideration?"

We made a rough estimate, based on some fantastic guesswork, of the number of women in the United States who might probably have a sincere desire for childbirth without any anesthesia. For reasons I can't remember we placed the figure somewhere over two million.

"Even supposing that's an exaggeration," I protested. "Why shouldn't those women be considered deserving of the same attention as the others? Now I see what's wrong with the course at the hospital; it's geared to the lowest common sensibility, to the most neurotic and fearful expectant mother. Granted that there should be a general education course for women who don't want anything more. Why not give the ones who do something satisfying?"

In answer Dr. Sedley pointed out some of the sad facts of money and personnel involved in giving even one course at the hospital. At the metalworkers' clinic in Paris all the women wanted the Pavlov method. At the average American hospital there were all sorts of women and all sorts of doctors. As for the private training I had had with Mme. Cohen, that would be financially unthinkable in America.

When I thought of the difference between the immense shining building of the American hospital and the modest old-fashioned cluster of buildings in Menilmontant I found it difficult to believe that the American institution was the poorer. When I thought of Mme. Cohen's sixth floor walk-up it was obvious that her financial reward was not very great. But I had to admit that if the Pavlov method were to be done in the United States it would have to be done on an American scale and that, like everything else, it would cost a lot of money.

Another time when I was complaining that much of the course at the hospital seemed to be bad conditioning rather than good, Dr. Sedley remarked, "When you use the word conditioning it sometimes sounds as though you mean repressing. From all you've said about it, the training you got in Paris sounds very dogmatic and doctrinaire. Americans don't take well to that sort of thing. You know what psycho-prophylactic means, don't you?"

I looked at him blankly. I didn't see what he was getting at

"Brainwashing," he said with a smile.

I thought about it a minute. "Well, why not?" I asked. "We're very scrupulous about washing everything else. Can you deny that our brains are a little muddy?"

"Can you deny the value of an open and free mind?" he said. "In this country we believe in letting people think for themselves. That's why the class is conducted as a discussion group."

"I never stopped thinking for myself during Mme. Cohen's course," I objected. "I didn't take anything on faith. I didn't have to—there was a good explanation given for everything. As for the brainwashing part, my mind became more free, not less, when it was emptied of destructive associations. As for the training's being doctrinaire, yes, it was doctrinaire and it worked. I was told to rehearse conscientiously and to expect that labor was going to be very hard work. I was assured that by using all the techniques I had learned I would be able to conquer pain. I wonder how many of the girls in that course who have been told just to relax and breathe deeply aren't going to be surprised when they discover what an overwhelming thing a powerful contraction is. I think the fact is that all those discussions of pain were just attempts to minimize the amount of pain there can be. The Pavlov method doesn't do that; it gives you tools with which to work."

"I must say," Dr. Sedley countered, "that it seems to me that very often Mme. Cohen presented what were only hypotheses as if they were thoroughly established facts. I don't think that's intellectually honest."

"Perhaps it wouldn't have been if her teaching had been purely informative," I said. "But as *training* I think it was fine.

I don't want to sound Pollyanna but it seems to me there is a power in positive thinking."

The tour of the hospital came two weeks later. I found it the most constructive part of the whole course. The delivery rooms at the Belvédère had been much like the labor rooms at this hospital (and indeed were used for both labor and delivery, a large operating room being reserved for emergencies). In comparison, the delivery room at the American hospital was at first big and frightening. When I walked in I had the feeling I had stepped into a science fiction film. But as soon as I got over being dazed by the impression that I was in a cave hung with gleaming metal objects, I realized that I was looking at a number of cabinets with glass fronts housing equipment of all sorts, metal cabinets on wheels (one of which turned out to be an electrically warmed cradle), a table full of tanks of anesthesia that looked like a miniature oil refinery, and a splendid metal and leather delivery table. At one end of the room was a glass-fronted gallery for students where we all sat while Miss Smiley demonstrated the workings of the delivery table. There were metal plates to which the legs were strapped, adjustable hand grips, and leather wrist thongs to keep the woman from reaching out and touching a sterile area. The bottom half of the table fell miraculously away and slid out of sight to give the doctor the best possible working position. Overhead was a great glaring dentist's light. "You'll quickly get used to that," Miss Smiley said.

When the demonstration was over we all came down and examined the table more closely. "How do they ever get you strapped into this fast enough?" I asked.

"You'll be wheeled in on the bed from the labor room and the nurses will take care of the rest," Miss Smiley said.

"Where's the mirror?" someone asked.

Miss Smiley reached up and pointed out the little round

mirror about six inches in diameter. "The nurse will adjust it so you can see what's happening," she said.

"Do we have to look?" someone asked.

"Not unless you want to," Miss Smiley answered turning it back up to the ceiling again.

"Oh, it's terribly exciting!" exclaimed the girl who had had natural childbirth before. "Of course, I didn't see the whole thing because the baby was so long in the birth canal they had to put me out and go after him with forceps, but just as soon as he was out, I came to and watched the doctor sew me up again. It was just fascinating! You can't imagine how interesting it was!"

"How long did he take to sew you up?" another girl asked.

"Oh, I was a special case—about forty-five minutes, but it didn't hurt at all."

"How many stitches did it take?"

And on and on they went.

I looked at the mirror. I tried to imagine what it would have been like if I had combined mirror watching with my pushing. The expulsion, as I remembered it, had required all my energy and concentration. If I had tried to watch myself perform, perhaps Dr. Lamaze would have had to go in and fetch the baby with forceps too. I must admit the mirror mania mystifies me. I'd much rather do something and do it well than see myself do it.

Someone asked to see a Trilene mask, and we all left the room discussing the offensive odor of Trilene. Just across the hall at the little round window of another delivery room was a nurse holding a newborn baby in her arms. We took turns peering at him through the window. The mother turned her head around and smiled at us from the delivery table. I was glad to be reminded that the ultimate purpose of all this shiny equipment was to bring such beautiful tiny human beings into the world.

The last meeting of the class was the husbands' session. We all sat around a table while our spouses made uncomfortable attempts at jokes. Miss Smiley ran through a little patter that put everyone at ease, and then we turned to the serious business of the evening. The husbands were invited to ask questions. But somehow they talked less than we women had and Miss Smiley was able to cover a lot of ground. She reviewed the first signs of labor and told us how to interpret them and when to start for the hospital. She explained the procedure when we got there, when the husband might join his wife in the labor room, where he could go during the delivery itself, and when he could see his wife again. She went on to a complete description of the stages of labor and what the husband could do to help his wife in each. I found it the best and most informative session of the course.

Miss Smiley was in the middle of repeating her amusing demonstration of pushing when the door opened and a young man stepped into the room. He stopped short, muttered, "I beg your pardon," and left, shutting the door behind him. A moment later it opened again and there he was, peering in at us.

"Are you looking for someone?" Miss Smiley asked.

"No," he answered. "That is, excuse me, but isn't this the motherhood course?"

"You might call it that."

"Well then, I just want to tell you all, I've been through this thing twice now and you ought to all pay attention to everything teacher says, and practice hard, and do your exercises, because it's wonderful, just wonderful!"

It was hard to say whether he was drunk or just overexcited. There were a few titters but mostly we just sat still, waiting for him to go away.

"My wife's up there right now," he said, taking two steps into the room. "Just had the second! A girl. That makes two girls!"

"Why don't you come in and tell us about it," Miss Smiley asked politely.

"I only want to tell you about this because I've been through it and I know what it's all about," he said, stepping into the room and loosening his collar. "It's the greatest! My wife took this course for the first one and she did fine. That's what I want to tell you. She really practiced the first time. This time, what with the other kid and the housework and just plain laziness, she didn't practice at all. Of course it was still pretty good, but she loused up the transition and she wasn't so hot in the delivery. But still it was the—"

"You weren't in the delivery room, were you?" one of the husbands cut in.

"No, they won't let you in the delivery room," he said. "But if you're nice to the nurses they'll sneak you down the hall and let you watch through the window in the door."

"Did you see the whole thing?"

"Except when someone stood in front of it. Believe me, I wouldn't miss it. But I'm gonna tell her next time not to be so sure, to stay in condition . . ."

He threatened to go on indefinitely. The atmosphere in the room was growing tense. It was obvious some of the people there did not appreciate his performance. Miss Smiley declared a coffee break.

When five minutes had passed and the young man had rushed off to see his wife, we returned to our places at the round table.

"Where were we now?" Miss Smiley asked.

We all thought a minute.

"Tell me one thing," one of the husbands asked slyly. "Was that rehearsed?"

Miss Smiley denied it vigorously, and we all laughed. But as far as I was concerned, it had been the most promising, positive note of the whole eight weeks.

9 Crise de Confiance

I had gone through the course at the hospital confident that I already knew about a way of giving birth that was more comprehensive and more effective than what was being taught there. I had marshaled my arguments in my discussions with Dr. Sedley with full faith that they were well founded. But now that it was over I suddenly began to feel the effects all this had had on me. A human mind does not work with the precision of a calculating machine. All conditioning is only temporary, and it may be modified and even eliminated by subsequent experience. This is, of course, the foundation of the attack on bad conditioning leading to pain that is so important in the Pavlov method. I now found that the same logic could apply to the conditioning of the method itself.

For sixteen hours I had sat talking about childbirth with seven other women and Miss Smiley. Of the nine of us, I and the girl who had had the Read training previously were the only ones who seemed to have a positive faith that childbirth could be a joyous instead of a painful experience. And there were elements in the story told by that other girl (her being put out, her forty-five-minute sewing up) that were not so positive either. The woman who had the caudals kept insisting that pain was inevitable. The other women didn't know. Their very uncertainty was somewhat contagious. And Miss Smiley, who very possibly has a great deal of faith in "natural childbirth," refused to commit herself on the subject of pain. It all depends on the individual was all she had to say.

Just about this time the article I had written so many months before was published by *Harper's Bazaar*. I read it through with the pleasant feeling that is always produced by seeing your own words in print, and patted myself on the back for having done my little bit to spread the good word. I was still enjoying that cozy feeling when I received a telegram forwarded by the magazine, from a woman in Illinois. "RE PAINLESS CHILDBIRTH JUNE ISSUE. WOULD APPRECIATE DETAILED REPORT ON EXERCISES AND IF POSSIBLE CHICAGO DOCTOR FAMILIAR WITH THIS METHOD. WOULD APPRECI-ATE INFORMATION FAST AS BEGINNING SEVENTH MONTH."

I stared at the telegram for a long time. Then I showed it to Alex and asked him what I ought to do. "I could translate Colette Jeanson, I suppose," I said at last, "but that would take too long. As for a doctor, I thought I'd made it clear that I hadn't heard of any doctor familiar with 'this method' in this country." I finally wrote her to try to find some place that did any kind of "natural childbirth" at all and suggested a few adaptations that might be helpful. I couldn't think of anything else to do—that was what I was doing myself.

Then the letters began to arrive. Now I know that letters written in response to an article in a magazine are more likely to be motivated by a gripe than by anything else. You have only to read the letter column in the *Times* every morning to see that people who are perfectly content with the world do not write. If I had received letters critical of what I had said about the Pavlov method, I don't think it would have bothered me. But the only such letter I got was from a woman in Trenton, N.J., who was disgusted with my being such a sissy as to need a *monitrice*. "I can deliver my own baby if I have to," she boasted, "*and* cut the cord." The others were either requests for more information, or letters from women who were interested in my article because they felt that in one way or another American doctors, hospitals, and courses in natural childbirth had let them down.

The requests for information were not discouraging, on the contrary. But they reminded me what a drop in the bucket my article was. Many of them were from doctors, one of whom complained that he had "heard snatches of the Pavlov method of delivery for quite some time" but to date had seen "nothing more official than an occasional reference to the fact that it is practiced extensively by the midwives of Russia." When it came to answering these requests I ran right smack into the language barrier. Of all the books I knew treating with the Pavlov method not a single one was in English. I sat down and wrote to Mme. Cohen asking her to keep me informed of anything that appeared on *Accouchement sans Douleur*. Then I answered the letters as best I could. But it was distressing being unable to satisfy the requests of doctors who wrote asking for something in English. One doctor can help so many women. All this served to remind me of the extent of the ignorance of the Pavlov method on this side of the ocean.

The effect of the other letters was more direct. Many of them were thoroughgoing horror stories. Some of them described experiences with natural childbirth only to point out the places where it had failed. Much of the blame for these failures was put on American hospitals and their way of treating women. One of these letters summed up many of the others. "Most American hospitals torture new mothers. They go on the theory that the hospital is there for the nursing staff and the doctors, not for the patient. The mother may be kept waiting half an hour while her history is recorded and certain assurances given that her bills will be paid. She is then stripped of her possessions, everything but her wedding ring, and hurried into a too-short, ugly hospital robe

. . . psychologically she is reduced to a nonentity, a person expected to react like a helpless baby, completely submissive. Treated this way, how can she be expected to participate fully in the birth process? All she wants is to be rendered unconscious of the terrors and encroaching discomforts. Insult is added to injury when she is put into a bed with bars like a crib. Treated like a rubber doll, how can she be meaningfully related to her normal life or her past?"

I was pretty sure none of this applied to my hospital. I had seen no beds with bars. Some of the letters confirmed my impression that it really was one of the places where a woman would be treated with consideration. But all the same, even with Dr. Sedley's support, I would be out if step with the system to some extent. He had pointed this out to me himself. I knew that many women in America had had very happy experiences with childbirth without anesthesia. But it was the letters from the others that I had read. I was struck by the fact that I was now in a similar situation to that of the women who had written me. I was on my own. This time I would have no team behind me. Mme. Cohen would not be there to help me through the difficult moments. Alex would do his best, but his experience was severely limited. Of course I had already had a successful delivery by the Pavlov method and I knew how to practice for it; I felt I could count on Dr. Sedley to ward off the anesthetist and to try to keep Alex with me the whole time, but all the same I could feel that the course at the hospital and the letters I had received had sown insidious seeds of doubt.

Each time I went to visit Dr. Sedley we discussed some aspect of what I was doing. He was always interested in what I had to say. He paid me the compliment of listening to me and of criticizing. "I wish you'd tell me a little more about what you did in France," he said. "And show me some of the exercises. I'd like to know more about what you're actually going to do."

I showed him a few of the limbering and relaxing exercises and then gave a demonstration of the way I had been taught to push.

"That's very interesting," he said. "But I don't see how that can make a particle of difference. Nature takes care of the pushing very nicely herself. It's an instinctive reflex. When the time comes, the woman just automatically bears down."

I hated to contradict him. He was the doctor after all. "It is an instinctive reflex," I agreed, "but it seems to me a woman can push more or less effectively. She can do things that interfere with the action of pushing or she can learn how to assist it. If she learns to wring the most out of each contraction, she can cut down on the amount of time the baby spends in the birth canal."

He looked at me skeptically. My certainty became a little less solid.

We talked about the breathing exercises. I explained that the breathing served the double purpose of creating a positive excitation in the cerebral cortex that inhibited the reception of pain and of increasing the supply of oxygen in the blood, which also eliminated pain.

"How?" he asked.

I did my best to reproduce what Mme. Cohen had said and what I had read in Colette Jeanson about the lack of oxygen and the accumulation of toxic substances in the uterus causing pain.

"That's all very interesting, Marjorie," Dr. Sedley replied. "But the whole theory of oxygen has not been proved. If it works for you, that's fine. Go ahead and use it. I'll be interested to see how you do."

I shrugged my shoulders. I was in no position to say anything more about such a technical matter.

"And what was this shot you say Mme. Cohen gave you?" he asked.

"Glucose," I said. "Its purpose was to restore my energy and wake me up."

"I wouldn't say that was a particularly tenable proposition either," he answered. "Although I don't doubt that it was psychologically helpful."

"You mean you think it was in just a sugar pill to help the hypochondriac?"

"Not that that can't have very real results." He smiled. "Most people are highly suggestible, and there's no question that the mind has a great influence on the body."

I certainly knew that. I was feeling highly suggestible then and there.

The next time I saw him was soon after my article appeared. As I was about to leave he commented that there were certain things m my article that he found shocking.

"What?" I asked, very much surprised.

"For instance, Mme. Cohen *threw* cold water in your face. I can promise that won't happen to you here. I confess that brutality of that kind shocks me. If anyone did a thing like that to one of my patients—"

"Perhaps I put it a little strongly in the article," I interrupted. "She didn't stand across the room and throw a bucket of water at me. She just gave my face and neck a good dousing with nice cold water. It wasn't brutal at all. It was just what I needed; stimulating and refreshing, especially as it was a warm summer night."

"Not everyone would react the way you did."

"Who knows? Perhaps Mme. Cohen would have thought of something else for another person." Then suddenly I thought of something. "Those are pretty fancy leather handcuffs on that delivery table," I said. "I hope it isn't an inflexible custom of the hospital to use them. That would be *my* idea of brutality."

"You can forget about them. I give you my word."

I walked home through the park pondering the idea that Dr. Sedley seemed to think of me as a nerveless amazon who enjoyed giving birth under conditions that were shockingly brutal. I knew the description didn't fit me. For the first time it crossed my mind that my first experience might have been a fluke.

The next thing to unnerve me was the question of the episiotomy. I hadn't had one in Paris because it hadn't been necessary. I had been able to keep from pushing while Dr. Lamaze delivered the baby with no ill effects either then or afterward. I had listened with some astonishment when the women in the course talked about the length of time it took them to get over their episiotomies. (One of them couldn't sit down for two weeks, the other occasionally felt pain nearly a year later—and I had always thought it was a matter of a few days.) Now suddenly Dr. Sedley began to tell me of the reasons why most American obstetricians performed episiotomies as a matter of routine. He explained that it was felt that the stretching of tissues, even if they did not tear, led to gynecological difficulties in later life. The episiotomy was done with a local anesthetic, he said, and was quite painless. He thought the women in the class must be exaggerating. He pointed out that an episiotomy was much neater than sewing up tears if they did occur. In spite of his arguments I decided to take the risk. Dr. Sedley agreed to go along with me if it was possible. I was grateful to him for leaving the decision up to me, as I think that is the sort of thing every woman has a right to decide for herself. But it did mean that there was one more obstacle to be hurdled.

The letters kept coming. "The next room contained a gal who shrieked all the time such pleasantries as 'God help me!' 'I can't stand the pain!' . . . A crew armed with pneumatic drills started repair work outside our wing at 8 A.M. . . . About an hour or two before delivery I overheard a nurse on the telephone say something about bringing the hearse around to the rear door." Friends told me bitter tales about how nasty nurses and obstetricians could be. One of them told me an incredible story of what had happened to her in one of the best hospitals in Philadelphia.

She had taken the course given at the hospital, practiced diligently, and turned up at the hospital feeling confident. Her doctor, a prominent member of the staff, had agreed to natural childbirth from the first. "As I was getting on toward transition he asked me if I wanted any anesthesia," she said. "I said I didn't. He cheerfully agreed that I wasn't to have any and then I saw him wink at the nurse. When I came to again it was all over." I got one letter from a woman who had been planning to have a caudal-forceps-episiotomy-mirror delivery (this too is called "natural childbirth") and had been put out totally when the lack of a mirror reduced her to tears. Of course it was easy to say "this won't happen to me," and rationally I had every reason to believe it wouldn't. But conditioning can be effected by irrational as well as by rational signals, and I could feel all this taking effect on me.

A book arrived in the mail from Paris. It was Dr. Vellay's *Témoignages sur L'Accouchement sans Douleur*. Turning the pages of the book the first thing I noticed was a whole series of fascinating pictures. Some of them were the very ones that had so upset me and then reassured me in Mme. Cohen's classes. For a few days I was too busy to read the book, but I occasionally glanced at the pictures and showed them to some friends. Their reactions varied widely. No one seemed upset by them as I had been, but some people did find it surprising that the women had let them be published. I took the book along on my next visit to Dr. Sedley and let him look at it. I was hoping the pictures might speak more eloquently for the Pavlov method than I had been able to. He glanced at them and then looked back at me a little strangely.

"What do you think of them, Marjorie?" he asked.

"I think they're extraordinary! I find them a real source of inspiration."

"Do you think the average woman would have the same reaction?"

"I don't know anything about the average woman," I said. "But I do know it was marvelous having them in my mind when the baby was being delivered."

"Don't you think they would be just as good if they had taken the trouble to blank out the faces?"

"I doubt it," I said. "The face tells the most important part of the story."

"Would you pose for such pictures?"

I felt myself blush. He made it sound like posing for dirty postcards. "I'm allergic to cameras," I said and dropped the subject. But what I thought was I wouldn't have the courage. And I was very thankful that those women *had* had it.

Dr. Sedley's reaction disturbed me. I began to realize the practical value of Mme. Cohen's repeatedly telling me *"C'est belle, n'est-ce pas? C'est belle!"* It wasn't that I actually thought that Dr. Sedley considered childbirth something shameful. But I had been made aware of the difference between the approach to the subject by Dr. Lamaze and Mme. Cohen, and the atmosphere that surrounds it in America. For instance, all that draping and wrapping in the examining and delivery room. I couldn't believe it was all for the purpose of sterility. I realized of course that lots of women have inhibitions—heaven knows I have plenty myself. But it seemed to me that this was an atmosphere that reinforced those inhibitions instead of encouraging a woman to get rid of them. I began to wonder if some of the attraction of anesthesia for both doctors and women didn't lie in the sop it offered to modesty. I began to see how Dr. Lamaze's assertion that the Pavlov method rendered the woman her full dignity as a human being had been thoroughly translated into practical and human terms in the way it was practiced in France.

None of these things was particularly important in itself, but the truth is that taken all together they had got me into a state where I really wondered if I could make a success of my approaching delivery. It did not seem that everyone could be out of step but me. The hymn to the highly differentiated individual offered me no comfort. My first delivery had not been easy. Second deliveries are supposed to be easier, but Dr. Sedley had explained that every delivery was an entirely different problem. I began to feel I had stuck my neck out by making all those assertions about the Pavlov method. Dr. Sedley, the nurses, my friends would all be interested to see if it would work a second time. I no longer was sure that it would myself, or that if I lost my control I wouldn't ask for the needle instead of trying to get the control back.

I was in the midst of brooding about all this when I got a letter from my friend who had borrowed the Colette Jeanson book months before. She wrote me to say that she had just had her baby, that she had followed all the instructions given in the book, and that it had been a tremendous success. "The most exciting moment was when the doctor suddenly shouted out, 'There now! He's spinning around now. Just look how he's spinning around!' I don't know why, but I felt such a sense of exaltation." Her letter gave me a tremendous lift. She had not studied with Mme. Cohen. It was her first child, and all she had to go by was the Colette Jeanson book. She had been successful in a situation that was roughly similar to mine, and with nothing to rely on but that.

A bit of my fighting spirit was restored when I ran into an old college friend who, sizing up my profile, dragged me into a bar and insisted on telling me the story of her delivery. The hospital where she lived gave no course in natural childbirth, so she had studied at home by reading Dr. Read's book. When labor started she was so relaxed that she waited around at home too long and nearly had the baby in the car. The minute she arrived at the hospital they rushed her straight to the delivery room. By the time she got on the table the baby was on his way out. An anesthetist tried to put a mask over her face in spite of her protests. When he attempted to force it on her, she took a jab at him in self-defense, and broke one of his teeth. At that moment the obstetrician arrived and delivered the baby while the nurses stood around and cheered. "I suppose it was the first natural childbirth they'd ever seen," she said. "Everyone was delighted—except the anesthetist of course. He wanted to sue me." Her means may have been rash, but then her situation was extreme, and I was proud of her.

Next I sat down and read Dr. Vellay's book. It turned out to be largely made up of excerpts from many of the reports that all women are asked to write after their deliveries. I found these wonderfully exciting reading, and the best possible answer to my uncertainties. There were examples of first births, second births, twins, breech deliveries, forceps deliveries (without anesthesia), induced labors, women who had had children by other methods before, women who were doctors or nurses, women with medical complications, women whose first children had been still-born, and many others. Each one reflected an individual personality in a way that was undeniably authentic. And again and again the Pavlov method worked for them. Even the chapter of cases considered to be failures proved encouraging—many of them would have been successes by any other standards. Included were women of many nationalities and reports from many countries—Italy, Belgium, Spain, Portugal, Switzerland, England, Russia, and China. I was delighted to discover the reports of three other American women who like me had had children in Paris by the Pavlov method. (One of them said, "*Accouchement sans Douleur* leaves you with a desire to have children for the pleasure of seeing them born.") I was also fascinated to discover that a Swiss obstetrician, Dr. Bonstein of Geneva, had spent some time at the University Hospital in Cleveland where he prepared and assisted at the delivery of twelve women with excellent results.*

* With the exception of this one program, which was abandoned shortly after Dr. Bonstein's departure as the result of the serious illness of the doctor who had planned to carry it on, I still know of no other place in the United States

Two of the reports of these women were reproduced in the book. One of them had previously had two children by "natural childbirth" with a caudal for the expulsion and said she very much preferred the Pavlov method. There could have been no more effective antidote for all the distressing tales that I had been exposed to.

Not long afterwards Mme. Cohen sent me a little review manual of the exercises and principles of the method, along with an encouraging letter telling me she was sure I would be able to make a success of my coming delivery. I immediately set about translating the manual so that I could send it to the women and doctors who had written to me for information. The tone was so straightforward, the directions so simple, and the explanations so logical that I immediately took Mme. Cohen's recommended practice outline as a guide and set about my own reconditioning.

Mme. Cohen also wrote me that an American woman whom she had prepared in Paris had found it necessary to return to America before her baby was due, and that I should soon hear from her. Not long afterwards I did get a letter from her, eight closely written pages sent from a Middle-Western city. I read it through once myself and then snatches of it aloud to Alex. "As you know I went to Mme. Cohen and I believe her faith in me and my ability to do it by myself, without having to transfer the responsibility to the *monitrice* played a great part in my success, because I certainly didn't get too much encouragement once I arrived in Denver. . . . My doctor was very nice about it in the

---

where the method is available. However, Dr. Lamaze told me in 1955 that an obstetrician from Philadelphia had come to Paris to spend several days studying at his clinic. In June, 1958, Dr. Vellay was invited to the *Congrès d'Obstétrique de Montréal* where *Accouchement sans Douleur* was one of the principal themes of discussion. Afterwards he made a short trip through several cities on the East Coast where he spoke to many obstetricians. In Montreal, he met one woman obstetrician who had come from the West Coast especially to learn about the Pavlov method. All of this makes one hopeful that before too long painless childbirth will be available to American women who want it.

fact that he said he would go along with me keeping the nurses with their hypos away from me and giving me oxygen instead of gas . . . but he said he didn't see much difference between this and the Read method and that a number of girls had wanted to try the Read method but that he'd never seen it work successfully. . . . Each one of my friends was skeptical, some said don't be surprised if your Dr. says he'll go along but then puts you under gas when the going gets tough and others saying not to set up such a mental block about this (i.e., that success or failure would mean that I was *personally* good or no good) so that I would feel guilty if I couldn't go through with it. They couldn't understand when I told them that if I ever admitted to the fact that I *might* take gas beforehand, it would be stupid to bother to try . . . I checked in at 6 . . . at ten minutes past six [the nurse] checked me and said I was dilated to three [centimeters] and then another nurse prepped me and gave me an enema and then the nurses left. The contractions were about two minutes apart by then but having just had all that soapy water poured in me I had to keep jumping up and running to the bathroom. This was bad because I'd invariably get caught having a contraction . . . by five of seven the contractions were fierce—pulling in front and back and the nurse checked me and said I was dilated to four. Then she went out. This was when it got hard. I was having very bad contractions and no one was in the room with me. The nurse having said I was at four had really lowered my morale because reasoning that I still had to go to ten for completion—I imagined another thirty minutes of this—I frankly didn't think I could stand it. I was panting loudly and heavily by this time and I remember a nurse coming in and saying 'What's wrong, what's wrong?' but I didn't even answer as I was concentrating so hard on my breathing . . . I had two contractions where I could feel the water nearly breaking and on the third it did and I felt the baby rush down. I yelled for someone and a nurse came in, took one look (she could see the head) and called for someone to get

Dr. Esmond—and then they wheeled me to the delivery room. They said don't push . . . so I figured I was in the transition period and panted and blew out. . . . This relieved me a lot. Then they made me climb on the delivery table and Dr. Esmond came in . . . but then every time I had a contraction and felt the urge to push he said to pant and relax (apparently the head was down to the perineum and he had to push against it with his fingers while I panted until the opening was enough and he could ease the head out). I then gave one more push and the baby was born. She cried and they laid her on my leg while they cut the cord. She really looked wonderful to me . . . I think that the French idea of (1) prepping yourself at home a few days before the due date, and of (2) taking a suppository or enema at home with the first contractions . . . of (3) going to the room and bed that you deliver in immediately on arrival at the hospital, and (4) of having someone with you to encourage and apprise you of what state you are in, might have made the difference between my five minutes of pain and what should have been five minutes more of hard work. This hospital is run like a factory. . . ."

When I read this letter for the first time I got the impression that she hadn't really been very successful. But going over it again it was obvious to me that her "failure" amounted to a victory over difficult circumstances. If she could do that well on her first try under those conditions, I was sure I ought to be able to be completely successful.

I put the letter in my pocketbook to serve as an inspirational talisman. That made two cases that I knew of personally where women had successfully had babies in American hospitals using the Pavlov method. And neither of them had had behind her the experience of a delivery in France. I suddenly realized that my goal ought to be not the mere repetition of my Paris experience but an altogether better one. "I'm going to prove to myself that the Pavlov method can be done with full success in this country,"

I told Alex. "From this moment on I refuse to discuss the possibility of failure. I'm determined to have a perfect delivery."

I increased my practice time. I cut down on the relaxing exercises which I found easy to do and concentrated on panting and preparing for the expulsion. It was obvious that I would have to be extra alert during the last phase. It didn't seem feasible to try to arrange the formal dialogue of direction that had been so carefully rehearsed in France. I would have to be so well prepared that I could ad-lib with skill. I made up my mind that I would cut down the time in the delivery room to an absolute minimum. I would make every push count for two!

As I exercised, I kept these resolutions in mind. I repeated each exercise, imagining that I was really in labor, and I concentrated as intently as I would have for the real thing. Unfortunately, I was carried away by my enthusiasm. I forgot all of Mme. Cohen's stern admonitions about moderation in the pushing exercise. I was thinking only of how I was going to make every push count as it had never counted before. And then suddenly I felt a spurt of water. I sat up, terrified. What had I done? There were still three weeks to go to my due date, and it seemed to me that I had burst the waters. I ran to the telephone and called Dr. Sedley.

"I think I've just broken the waters," I told him nervously. "What should I do about it?"

"Are you sure it was amniotic fluid?" he asked calmly.

"I think so."

"What were you doing at the time?"

"Exercising. Excessively." I felt terribly stupid.

"Nothing to worry about. Just call me and let me know if you lose any more."

I waited anxiously the few days till my next office visit. When he had completed his examination, Dr. Sedley asked calmly when I would like to have the baby. The question startled me. "Naturally I'd like to have it as soon as possible," I said.

He looked at me thoughtfully. "Would you prefer Tuesday or Friday?"

"Why? Are you in direct communication with the higher powers?"

"You know, Marjorie," he said, "we could induce labor any time next week. The cervix is completely effaced—dilatation of two centimeters, and the baby is a pretty good size. I'm in favor of inducing myself. The labor will be much shorter."

"But induced labors are much harder to control, aren't they?" I asked. "They proceed so rapidly. I read about one in Dr. Vellay's book. The woman said the contractions kept surprising her."

"I don't think there's that much difference," Dr. Sedley replied.

I was still concerned about the water I had lost. Dr. Sedley didn't seem to think it was a significant amount if, indeed, I had lost any at all. Then I thought about having the baby. After all those months I wanted to learn who was inside there. The idea of picking out a birthday and giving birth on it was mighty tempting, and Dr. Sedley thought it was a good idea. I agreed to the induction. We set the date for Tuesday, the seventeenth. I was confident that if I went on practicing, this time with discretion, and rested well the night before, no matter how fast the contractions mounted in intensity I would be able to deliver this child in full control.

10 *It's a Girl!*

I counted off the days, each morning knowing that I could still call Dr. Sedley and change my mind. I was torn between my natural desire to have the baby and the superstitious feeling that nature ought to choose the moment when a child comes into the world. I half hoped the baby would arrive of its own accord before the date we had agreed on. I took long, long walks, which actually did stimulate contractions of a feeble sort. Unfortunately they stopped every time shortly after I finished my walk.

The night before my appointment at the hospital, Alex and I went to an excellent Chinese restaurant. We lingered over a well-proportioned and delectable feast, feeling comfortably smug in the idea that we were about to behave with very good sense. Unlike the last time, I would go to bed early, awaken from a night of refreshing sleep, and go to the hospital in a state of full vigor and alertness. On the way home we talked about how amazing it was that the next day an entirely new person would have come into the world. I was filled with this kind of happy anticipation right up to the moment when I snuggled down for that long night of salutary sleep.

I did a quick mental review of the techniques of the method, thinking that it was a good thing to have that be the last impression on my mind before I fell asleep. That trick had always brought me excellent results in examinations at school. This time it turned out merely to be the springboard for one of those nightlong dialogues that turn up the same ideas again and again as though they were something discovered for the first time. I caught a little sleep toward morning, and awoke not much more rested than I had gone to bed. I wonder if it is ever possible to start labor in that recommended state of dazzling freshness.

Still, there it was at last—Tuesday morning, September the seventeenth, the day I was going to have the baby! A fine sooty rain was making a pleasant drumming on the air-conditioner. I was just beginning to wish I could curl up and spend the day in bed when the alarm began to buzz. "Can't be late today!" I said, poking Alex in the ribs and suddenly found myself leaping out of bed. I stood in the middle of the room for a minute wondering what to do next. The whole situation suddenly seemed improbable. I thought about what to wear, and then remembered that it didn't much matter. I got back into the clothes I had worn the night before while Alex made some coffee. Then I placed my suitcase squarely in front of the door so I couldn't possibly forget it and joined Alex in the kitchen. We swallowed the coffee, put on our raincoats, and silently left, leaving the apartment still dark and asleep.

We made the classic picture as we stood on the wet sidewalk and waited for a stray taxicab. Classic that is, except that there was no labor. I began to feel it was all a huge practical joke. I imagined a scene where we were met at the hospital door by a startled nurse who stared at us blankly and then in answer to my awkward attempts to explain snapped coldly, "Nonsense! What nonsense! No labor, no baby."

It turned out that the world is much more used to such occurrences than I had thought. A taxi came along and the driver even refrained from any comments—the first one to do so in weeks. The receptionist only nodded when I gave my name. She typed out a little card for the files and then escorted us to the elevator.

The room on the seventh floor was pleasantly remote from the world. Alex and I sat and looked at each other. There was nothing to say. We opened books, but it was difficult to concentrate. I put on the little hospital gown that was waiting for me and sat down on the bed. Alex said it looked very chic, but I presume that was meant only by way of conversation.

Nothing happened for some time. Once someone popped a head in and looked surprised to see us. "Oh, you're here?" she said. "How are your pains?"

"I'm not having any," I answered, feeling a little foolish.

"Oh," she said, and vanished. It idly went through my head that it was supposed to be psychologically bad practice to ask about "pains," but by this time I was so thoroughly acquainted with the question that even my intellectual interest was very mild.

We had arrived promptly at eight; it was now after nine. I had finally decided that the doctor must have had an emergency call elsewhere when a nurse marched in the door to do the preparation. She asked Alex if he wouldn't like to step outside for a cigarette. He blankly answered that he didn't smoke. I had forgotten to warn him that in America the husband is constantly being sent out for a smoke. "Yes, darling, why don't you go have a cigarette?" I urged.

"There's a nice waiting room just down the hall to the right," the nurse explained delicately. Alex finally got the idea and departed.

The prepping was carried out in a pleasantly deft manner. The nurse was a paragon of gentleness and consideration. After all the complaints I had heard about the unpleasantness of hospital prepping, I was delighted. Then it occurred to me that I was not in labor, and that that might make all the difference. It might be quite another experience coming in the middle of a contraction. The nurse stayed to chat awhile until Alex came back from the waiting room. Then she left us to wait some more.

A resident physician dropped around to ask the routine questions. A lot of them seemed terribly unnecessary, and my answers were perfunctory. It wasn't till he left that I began to wonder if they hadn't been so perfunctory as to be inaccurate. Looking back over my limited hospital experience I can't remember ever having given a resident physician a straight story. There is something about them that makes me want to list an extra grandmother on the paternal side or say I had twin aunts who died of hiccups. For all their gravity I had the impression that they are superfluous. A nurse has just taken your blood pressure and written it down, when one of them marches in, takes it again, and writes it down again. Two minutes later the doctor arrives. He does not look at what the others have written but takes it a third time. Nor does he write it down. This gives you plenty to think about.

In the midst of this harmless speculation Dr. Sedley arrived with the intern trailing along after him. We passed the time of day for a few minutes, and as they left I gathered from their conversation that I had been granted an appointment on the ninth floor at eleven o'clock for the purpose of rupturing the membranes.

At five of eleven we marched down the corridor to the elevator. We made a charming procession, a nurse at the head, looking official, me behind in my fetching hospital robe, and Alex bringing up the rear with his book in one hand and my powder and sponge in the other. We stepped out on the ninth floor and stood waiting awkwardly in the corridor. They were having a busy morning and they hadn't quite decided where to fit us in. At that Alex opened his book and began to read. He can read in the midst of anything.

At last they were ready for us. Alex was sent out for another smoke and the nurse outlined the procedure. The doctor would rupture the membranes in one of the delivery rooms after which we would all move into a labor room. I shuffled along after her to a delivery room where I shed my paper slippers and was maneuvered into position on the fancy table. For the first time I got into those funny white leggings that one sees in pictures of deliveries. I had always imagined they were part of the sterility measures but the nurse said they were to protect my legs from the cold metal. After she had strapped me into the stirrups she set about adjusting them to a nice even position. "A little lower?" she asked, fiddling with the assorted screws and bolts. "No, no, but more to the right," I answered. It was rather like hanging a picture. "Do we go through this again during the delivery?" I asked. "Don't worry about that," she answered cheerfully. "It doesn't take any time at all."

The entrance of Dr. Sedley and the intern spared me any further consideration of the subject. They set right to work on the rupturing. The nurse began the ceremony by baptizing me with what seemed to be at least a gallon of icy pink solution. This little ritual was to recur very frequently right up to the expulsion of the baby. Every time I commented on the chilly temperature of the water I was informed that it was actually at body temperature. The rupturing itself was not quite the rapid sensationless puncturing that I had expected from Mme. Cohen's description given over two years before. Instead it felt like a long examination with a lot of poking, twisting and pushing, during which it took all my concentration to remain relaxed. I tried to remember the appearance of the puncturing gadget I had seen at the Belvedere and to form some picture in my mind of what was going on. I find that a good mental image is almost always an effective tool against tension. Finally it was over and the nurse began detaching me from the armor.

I lay there waiting while the three of them discussed the relative merits of one brand of something or other over another. Dr. Sedley defended his choice on the grounds that it was made up of natural rather than synthetic ingredients. I was just thinking how much I approved of his reasons, when I realized that the product in question was something he was about to inject into my arm. "Help!" I said, terrified by the sight of the needle. "What's that?"

Dr. Sedley patiently explained that it was a necessary part of inducing labor. From time to time he was going to give me small amounts of oxytocin, a hormone extract from the posterior pituitary gland that stimulated uterine contractions. It occurred to me how ridiculous I was to have seriously thought I could get in and out of a hospital without being stuck with a needle.

"We'll go to the labor room now," the nurse said, when the injection was over. I started to get up. "No, no," she stopped me. "Don't get up. Just slide over onto this bed and travel in style." I was just about to protest that I was not an invalid, when I felt my uterus pull up into a great, taut mound, and stay there. Is this the first contraction? I wondered. It wasn't like any of the contractions I had had before. It didn't begin slowly, then rise to a peak, then fade away. It just appeared, a big hard lump, and stayed. It astonished me to think that a shot in the arm could bring on a contraction so quickly. For the first time it occurred to me that induced labor might not follow the pattern I had been taught to expect.

I remembered a sentence from Mme. Cohen's manual. "The different stages of labor may occur more quickly than you expected, and the alert mind of a well-trained woman must adapt itself immediately to each situation." It was clear that the first thing to do was to try to analyze the contractions so as to be able to anticipate their behavior. I reached under the sheet and placed my hands lightly on my abdomen. I felt the uterus soften and return to normal. In less than a minute, however, it had pulled up taut again. The contraction was very weak, but it lasted a long time.

I began to do deep, slow breathing and a very light *effleurage* as a kind of anticipatory insurance. It turned out to have an excellent effect. Doing the familiar rhythmic breathing was calming and reassuring. As long as my hands were on my abdomen, I knew that there was no chance that a contraction would catch me unaware. I felt a little conspicuous rolling down the corridor with what I thought must be a glassy stare of Pavlovian concentration, but I didn't much care.

By the time I was established in my labor room I had experienced at least three such contractions and it seemed that the pauses between them were lengthening. I asked the nurse for something to put under my knees. She immediately produced a blanket from somewhere and rolled it up and put it under my legs. Unfortunately it was not quite long enough so that one leg or the other was constantly sliding off to the side. When Alex came back I asked him to reroll it. This time one end was higher than the other and I listed a little to starboard. He rerolled it and I listed to port. It was just like being on a camping trip and trying to find a really level spot for your sleeping bag. Still, it had the advantage of keeping Alex from being bored. Every fifteen or twenty minutes he could readjust the blanket roll.

No sooner was I comfortably settled than Dr. Sedley reappeared. "How are you doing?" he asked. I had to confess that nothing much was happening. Whereupon he got out the needle again and injected another dose of that non-synthetic oxytocin preparation. Just then I noticed a large bottle that stood on the table by the wall.

"You aren't planning to pump all of that into my arm?" I asked warily. His only answer was a noncommittal laugh.

Almost immediately the contractions picked up with redoubled force; again there was very little time in between. I began to breathe as deeply as possible. Dr. Sedley watched me with interest. "How long do you suppose it will be until the baby is born?" I asked when the contraction was over, trying to sound as nonchalant as possible.

"Oh, an hour or two," he answered casually. I couldn't tell whether he was joking or not. Compared to my first delivery that seemed incredible. Alex went off again to get costumed properly, and Dr. Sedley went to look in on another patient. The contractions had become more regular and much more intense. The time between them had lengthened to what seemed to be about three minutes. I kept very comfortably in control of them by doing the *effleurage* and the deep and slow breathing. My only concern was that if they got much stronger I might be forced to switch to the rapid superficial breathing. Since I didn't really believe that labor could be so short, it seemed a little early for that.

Every few minutes a nurse would peek in to see how I was coming along. It was nice knowing that I hadn't been forgotten, but it was a little disconcerting to my concentration. For example: a contraction had just got under way. I had been alert, caught it at the very beginning, begun the *effleurage* and breathing in plenty of time, and was following its course uphill toward the peak when—the door opened. A bright pretty face looked in at me and a cheery voice said, "Hello there! How are you? Who do you think is leading at the Polo Grounds?" Normally I would have answered something like "Fine thanks! Who's playing?" But if I said even that now, I might fall behind the contraction. So I was forced to be rude. I went on massaging with one hand and held up the other, finger pointed, in a gesture that I hoped would be interpreted as a request to wait. But by the time the contraction had subsided the face had disappeared again.

Alex came back. He handed me the talc from time to time, but there was nothing much more for him to do. They had given him a pretty white hospital outfit, and he was looking immensely pleased with himself. He proudly pointed out a little attachment he was wearing on the soles of his shoes. It was to ground him in the delivery room, he explained. Apparently there is so much equipment in the delivery room that if you aren't properly grounded you are likely to be electrocuted. "Don't worry," he said, "you won't ever touch the ground." The whole idea delighted him; it horrified me.

Dr. Sedley was back again. I was beginning to wonder if he would go away again without giving me another shot if I said the contractions were tremendous. I brooded over this question for some time. Later on I realized that he was probably giving me the shots on a schedule, and it wouldn't have made any difference what I said.

Things began to move ahead much more rapidly. I had to switch over to panting, and my tolerance for jokes and conversation about the weather dropped off sharply. I stopped caring whether or not people thought I was rude. I stopped holding my finger up for silence, and simply relied on a sharp hiss and Alex's explanations. Even that consisted mostly of "Wait till the contraction's over." He also asked the nurses to listen to the foetal heartbeats only in the moments between contractions.

About this time people began to ask me solicitously if I wouldn't like "a little something to take the edge off." I don't know if my panting looked like a sign of suffering or if it was just a routine offer. I had the impression that they considered it a moral duty to keep reminding you that they could ease your sufferings whenever you needed relief. Actually I am certain that almost any woman in labor is capable of shouting for something if she really wants it. At least, judging from the moans and pleas that drifted in whenever the door was open, women in labor are not shy. By concentrating, panting, and doing the *effleurage*, I was riding safely on top of the contractions. It was beginning to be hard work, but their offers were about as tempting as a glass of fish oil.

Each time I began to feel overconfident, Dr. Sedley returned with another shot. Off the contractions raced, and off I went after them. They were mounting steeply, but just as I was afraid that they might get out of hand, they tapered sharply and were gone. I found that it was more restful to pant only up to the peak and then drop back to the slow, deep breathing. The *effleurage* was still very helpful. I'm afraid that at the peaks my breathing was no longer beautiful, silent, and rhythmic. But it was marvelously effective all the same.

About this time I had my first encounter with differences of technique. A nurse walked in and saw me panting and massaging. A look of deep sympathy swept over her face. "There, there, dear," she said. "Just let your hands drop limply at your sides, breathe deeply way down into your tummy, and relax." Fortunately Alex told her that I was doing it my own way, and she left. I was beginning to get positively intolerant, not only of advice but of jokes and small talk, indeed of anything that might interfere with my concentration.

I was well into the second hour of labor when I experienced a discomfort quite unlike anything I had felt before. Perhaps it was related to the sensation that is known as back labor, but actually it felt more like side labor, if there is such a thing. Massage didn't do very much good. I turned on my side which seemed to relieve it, but Dr. Sedley asked me to get back on my back as the side position seemed to be slowing up the contractions. Fortunately it was only a minor irritation.

The contractions had become very strong. I was quite cantankerous about making nurses wait till they were over to listen to the foetal heartbeat. Then a new nurse wandered in to take her crack at me. She had short red hair and a delicate twinkle in her eye. Seeing that I was doing some sort of activity of my own, she stood by the bed and waited until the contraction in progress was over. "Well," she said to Alex. "Just look at that! She seems to have worked out a little system all her own. She's patting her tummy and panting like a puppy. Look," she added to Dr. Sedley who had just come in. "She's patting her tummy and panting like a puppy, and it seems to do her good!" She was the first person who had noticed what I was doing and the effect it had before leaping in with routine suggestions of her own. She was someone I should have liked to see more of.

Suddenly an absurd thing happened. Between contractions

I found myself shaking in a most alarming manner. My teeth chattered loudly; my arms and legs seemed about to fly off by themselves. It was not painful but it made me afraid that I would miss the beginning of a contraction and lose control. Alex offered to try to hold my legs still, but they jumped around despite his grasp on them and the restraint gave me a feeling of terrible nervousness. A nurse who looked in told me that this was a fairly common phenomenon. Fortunately it turned out that the moment I began to pant the trembling stopped completely and only resumed when the contraction was over. I wondered if it were not some sort of automatic release of stored-up tension, because once I got used to the idea, the shaking was almost pleasurable. But it did mean I had to work even harder on concentrating.

Dr. Sedley sent Alex out for another smoke, and proceeded to examine me. In the course of his probing I found myself nearly overwhelmed by a violent contraction. In spite of myself I became tense and made a lot of noise huffing and puffing. I felt I was losing control when I heard Dr. Sedley say something about the dilatation. The word made a sudden mental image in my mind. "Dilatation." There was the baby's head pressing down on a ring that had stretched to a diameter of eight centimeters. As the contraction mounted in force I imagined the ring being pulled open larger and larger. As I watched this work being accomplished in my imagination, the threat of pain vanished. When the examination was over, Dr. Sedley predicted it would be only another half hour or so for the dilatation to be complete. This was vastly encouraging news. When the next contraction came, I experimented with my new discovery. As long as I went on visualizing what was happening my control was perfectly secure; as soon as I lost the mental image the force of the contraction began to threaten me. I was so elated by that discovery that I felt that I could carry on for hours more, if necessary.

A few contractions came and went and a new nurse entered the room. "Relax," she commanded, after the most fleeting glance in my direction. "Try to relax and breathe deeply with the abdomen —like this." I almost laughed, the thought of abdominal breathing was so impossible. Then suddenly I had what struck me as a funny feeling. Something made me think that the baby had dropped through the cervix. Certainly not more than ten minutes of the half hour Dr. Sedley had predicted for me had passed, and I didn't feel any wild desire to push. Still, it was a peculiar sensation, and I thought I'd better mention it to the nurse. She immediately rushed out to find the doctor.

What followed was a scene of almost classic confusion. The nurse came back with the young intern in tow. For some reason he pulled my bed out from the wall. Some other people popped in and out, all talking at once. Someone asked in a joking tone if I'd mind terribly having my baby in the labor room as none of the delivery rooms was free at the moment. There was a grim edge to the voice that indicated it wasn't really a joke at all. I couldn't have cared less. Suddenly my only interest had become getting permission to push.

"Certainly," I answered, "only get my husband in here and tell me if it's all right to push now."

No one paid attention to my little speech. Most of it was drowned in the general confusion. The desire to push was fast becoming urgent. I blew out forcefully a couple of times, and panted a little in between. I really hadn't much idea of what they all were doing. I had to mark time somehow, and I was succeeding.

Dr. Sedley appeared in the doorway and asked me if I would mind having the baby in the labor room.

"Not at all," I repeated, "but may I please push now?"

"Ha! Ha! He isn't joking!" someone said.

I wasn't joking either. I pulled at the intern's sleeve and repeated my request. For the first time he appeared to be aware of my existence.

"What is it?" he asked.

"May I push now?"

"What? Oh yes, go ahead."

That was all I needed to hear. I took a deep breath, blew it out, took another and held it. I began to push. I didn't push unduly hard—I was in no great hurry to expel the baby until they had decided which room they preferred. I discovered that there was a point at which I felt superbly comfortable and happy, and beyond which there was no need to push unless I wanted to. So I just pushed to that pleasant point and waited happily while everyone conferred. As I felt the desire to push grow stronger, I increased the force of my push just enough to keep feeling happy. I was confident that if the baby actually began to come out they would all quiet down and help.

From somewhere down the hall came the cry of a new baby. It gave me a tremendous feeling of elation. I felt marvelous. That seemed to be the signal to set me rolling. Dr. Sedley walked beside my bed. He talked to me slowly, clearly and distinctly, as if, for some reason, he thought I couldn't hear him. Or maybe it just seemed that way to me. "Are you sure you want me to deliver the baby without an episiotomy?" he asked.

"Yes," I answered somewhat impatiently. It seemed to me the question had been settled.

"Then I'll do it without one," he answered. "I expect you to give me your complete cooperation."

I thanked him and promised to do my best. They started to push me down the corridor. Alex joined the cortege. I greeted him briefly and went on pushing. I could feel the baby moving along, and I was wonderfully happy. The clock in the delivery room said 2:40 as we entered. I didn't want to waste another minute.

I was surprised to find the stirrup adjustment was much easier than it had been earlier. Dr. Sedley was in the corner washing his hands. The anesthetist was behind the table. The intern was fussing with the little mirror that hangs near the light. "Can you see?" he asked me.

"What?" I answered.

"What way would you like the mirror turned?"

"I don't want any mirror," I said. "I just want to have my baby." He looked at me dubiously, and turned the mirror to the ceiling. I'm sure he found me wanting in intellectual curiosity.

I felt another urge to push. I inhaled, exhaled, inhaled, held, and this time really leaned into it. The nurse who previously had instructed me to breathe abdominally began a little speech about bearing down, but after a few words she stopped and said, "Well, well, she does know how to push!" (All through the expulsion people referred to me as though I weren't actually there. I felt a little like an eavesdropper.)

The anesthetist asked me if I wanted something "to take the edge off." The contraction was finished and I felt very relaxed and as though I had all the time in the world to talk.

"What do you have?" I asked, wondering if she was going to offer me oxygen. It was like the "What do you have?" that I use to learn about the possibilities of the liquor closet when I know perfectly well that whatever there is I'll have a bourbon.

"How about some nitrous oxide?" the anesthetist suggested.

"No, thanks," I said. "I don't want anything."

The next contraction came. I took a deep breath and pushed as hard as I could. In the middle of the contraction Alex had to remind me to take in more air. I was so intent on pushing that I quite forgot. When the contraction was over we waited in silence. It was delightfully restful to have that moment of absolute quiet. Nobody thought of spoiling it with friendly chatter.

On the next contraction there was a minor crisis. I pulled so hard on the hand grip that it came loose and slid up the side of the table. "Will somebody fix this damn thing!" I exclaimed. The anesthetist was the first person to see what had happened. She quickly shoved the grip back in place and screwed it down again. I was very pleased to have had her there.

Another push. Suddenly Dr. Sedley's voice said, "Stop pushing." I stopped and began to pant. He manipulated the baby's head while the nurse put her hand on my abdomen. Then I heard him say, "Push down." Almost automatically, I did so.

"She's pushing, I think," the intern said a moment later.

"Stop pushing," Alex told me. I stopped again.

"Push down over here," Dr. Sedley said again. I didn't quite understand what he meant, so I pushed very tentatively. "Push down here," he repeated.

"She's pushing again," the intern said.

"What do they want?" I asked Alex.

"Just relax," he said. "Pant." I did so.

"Push," Dr. Sedley said.

"He's talking to the nurse," Alex explained. So that was it! Once I realized what was going on, I relaxed and waited for the baby to be delivered. It was done with marvelous skill and delicacy. I felt the head come out and then the shoulders. Then he held her up in the air. She began to cry. She didn't say, "La!" because it wasn't France. She sang out with a very penetrating "Waaaa!" There she was! Marianne Margaret! The nurse put her down on top of me half wrapped in sterile sheets. I held her precariously by one arm. I was so amazed by the discovery that she didn't look anything like Pepi that I nearly dropped her. The cord was cut, and then the intern snatched her away again and started to put drops in her eyes.

"Push again, Marjorie," Dr. Sedley commanded.

"What?" I asked stupidly. "What for?"

"The placenta," he answered. I had forgotten all about it in my excitement. It came out in one push. Dr. Sedley examined it, seemed satisfied, and went to wash his hands. "Congratulations!" he said, shaking hands with Alex. Then he dashed out of the room before I had a chance to thank him. "He has another patient across the hall," the nurse explained. "She chose the same moment you did to produce."

The nurse reminded me that I would have to spend the next hour in the delivery room under observation—standard practice. She showed me the placenta and the intern asked me more questions and filled out a little chart with the answers. He told me the moment of birth had been 2:59. That was something I would never have believed earlier in the day. It had been 11:30 by the time they had ruptured the membranes. The whole process had taken only three and a half hours.

Marianne was lying in the electrically warmed cradle at the side of the room. I couldn't wait to have another good look at her. I asked the nurse if I could see her, and she picked her up and brought her over to me. She seemed bigger than Pepi had been, even though she had come earlier (actually she did weigh a pound more than he had). Alex stood next to me and we both stared at her looking for family resemblances. Then the nurse put her back in the cradle.

I was impatient at having to lie there on the delivery table. I had never felt better in my life. All I wanted to do was have a big lunch and call my mother to tell her how splendid life was.

Alex and I looked at each other and laughed. "There you are," he said. "The Pavlov method works in America too."

"It certainly does," I answered. "But I'm starved. Why don't you go out and get me a chocolate milkshake?"

And he did.

Afterword by Alex Karmel

Philippa has always been somewhat jealous about being left out of her mother's book, and for good reason. The circumstances of her delivery were at least as interesting as those of her brother and sister, and again a tribute to the effectiveness of the Lamaze method. By 1960, when Philippa was born, Marjie had already begun the efforts that led to the founding of the American Society for Psychoprophylaxis in Obstetrics (ASPO). This time around our obstetrician, one of the founders of ASPO, was enthusiastic. It seemed assured that everything would go smoothly. But then it happened that Philippa arrived a month early and, moreover, was a breech baby.

If Marjie's doctor was on her side, the hospital where Philippa was born gave us enough opposition to create a drama. Marjie's contractions began unexpectedly at midnight while we were talking with two close friends after a good dinner at a restaurant. Having the experience of two births behind her, Marjie knew this was the real thing. We called the obstetrician and took a cab to the hospital. As so often happens, there were many papers to be filled out first, but after a while she had a room. She was barely installed, her clothes in the closet and her toilet case over the sink, when the doctor, having driven in from the suburbs, arrived to examine her.

He confirmed what Marjie had already sensed: Birth was imminent.

Marjie was already using all the skills she had learned to keep in control. It was now two in the morning. For some reason or other, the only delivery room available was a grand amphitheater, so that is where we went. The obstetrician hurriedly threw a white gown over my shoulders and gave me a surgical mask. "Say you're a doctor," he advised me. "Any kind of doctor!"

We already knew that the hospital was not accustomed to fathers being present during deliveries; now we learned that the chief nurse had said she would leave if ever a father was admitted to a delivery room. And that is just what happened. As soon as Marjie, now on a rolling table, our doctor and I walked into the amphitheater, the chief nurse took off her hat and apron and walked out. It didn't matter to us; there were other nurses who stayed.

What was important was the intense dialogue that took place between Marjie and her physician, all through the hour that followed. A breech delivery is not like the usual delivery; in a sense everything is in reverse order so far as the child is concerned. I do not think that Marjie could have done it if Philippa had been her first child, but because of her training and experience she was able to follow directions about when to push, when to push a little, and when to stop pushing altogether—all this in opposition to the signals to bear down constantly that her body was sending her. It is certain that, if she had been given any anesthesia, she couldn't have done it. But in any event, things went so fast that drugs wouldn't have had time to take effect, had she desired them.

Of all three, this was the delivery that demanded the most of Marjie as a controlled, conscious mother, but it was also the one during which she felt the least threatened by pain. I was at her side, telling her that she was doing very well; the doctor gave instructions which she followed. The experience was so intense that none of us was aware of anything else.

In the meantime, word had gone out that there was a breech delivery in progress without anesthesia, the first, perhaps, in that hospital, in fifty years. The result—it was now almost three in the morning—was that the ranks of seats reserved for spectators rapidly filled up with nurses, doctors, interns, orderlies, and aides, including the chief nurse who had so dramatically left the operating floor. This created an audience for Philippa's theatrical arrival. Marjie greatly enjoyed hearing about it later; while it was going on she was too busy to notice anything aside from what she was doing.

What she was doing was giving birth to our second daughter, and we both knew early in the process that it was a girl, because what came out first was a couple of dark-purple minuscule legs, followed by two tiny buttocks. The hard part, demanding skill on the part of both obstetrician and mother, was the delivery of the arms, then the shoulders, and, most critical of all, the head. But by then, I think, the drama of the situation, and perhaps even some awareness of the audience, helped Marjie a bit. She was an actress by profession; she got into the business of telling women and men about a more human way to have their children very much by accident.

After some delicate manipulation, the head was delivered and the usual ritual of cutting the cord followed. No longer having to concentrate, Marjie was exhilarated. Philippa was weighed and found to be just a gram above having to be put in an incubator; instead, she was put into her mother's arms.

Since Philippa's head had come out chin first, her face was not at all wrinkled; she was the most beautiful newborn baby I had ever seen. (Some of that delicacy, I think, continues to this day, but I will let her friends judge for themselves.)

What is lacking in my postscript is what Majorie Karmel would have written about her own experience of this remarkable occasion. Her tragic death arrived before she got around to it, and before she got around to so many other things she would have done, many of them not at all related to the subject of the book you have been reading.

A Lamaze Manual
for the '80s

BY MARILYN FREEDMAN

NOTE: The following guide is not intended to take the place of childbirth preparation classes, nor does it pretend to offer a comprehensive practical manual; there are books listed under "Suggested Reading" that cover the subject more fully. Offered here is, rather, a basic summary of the Lamaze method of prepared childbirth as it has evolved during the years since *Thank You, Dr. Lamaze* was first published.

The author, Marilyn Freedman, is a registered Physical Therapist and a certified Childbirth Educator through ASPO, the American Society for Psychoprophylaxis in Obstetrics, Inc. She is past president of the Long Island chapter of ASPO in New York and currently has a private practice in childbirth education, pre- and postnatal exercises, and physical therapy. She is also a childbirth consultant on the advisory board of *American Mother* magazine.

Childbirth preparation is an adventure in self-mastery. Ideally the program should begin long before conception, be augmented and intensified during the last eight to twelve weeks of pregnancy, and continue into the postpartum period. Essential to it is an understanding of good nutrition and the living patterns conducive to a healthy body. It is now known that smoking, drugs, and alcohol can be harmful to the unborn child. Eating sensibly, alleviating stress, learning to make choices for yourself—all are critical factors during the year your baby is born.

Phase I

The first phase of the program is designed to produce the relaxation, body awareness, and body conditioning that will enable you to use the specific tools you will later develop for the optimum labor and birth experience.

Relaxation and Body Awareness

"*Nesting*": Settle yourself in a comfortable position, sitting, lying, or half reclining on your back or side. Your arms and legs should be independently supported, their joints in mid-flex (neither fully bent nor fully extended) with the help of pillows, rolled-up blankets, or towels.

Breathing: Notice your breathing. Is it rhythmical? deep? shallow? Through your nose? your mouth? Does your rate of breathing change when you are tense or afraid, excited or sad? Your awareness of the importance of uninterrupted breathing, whether shallow or deep, will help you in the stress of labor later.

Before starting any of the exercises that follow, take one or more deep breaths in and out. In Lamaze (as in yoga) these are spoken of as "cleansing breaths," but many childbirth educators call them *greeting breaths* since they are used preceding each activity/exercise/contraction. Complete each activity with another cleansing breath, called here *completion breath*. Take a deep breath in through your nose, expanding your chest, and then relax, exhaling through slightly parted lips. Do this a few times and then allow your breathing to find its natural rhythm.

TUNING THE REST OF YOUR BODY TO AWARENESS

These exercises, done in your favorite nesting position, will enable you to distinguish between areas of tension and relaxation and learn how to release any residual tension. This is as important during pregnancy, with its added stresses and strains, as it is in labor and delivery, when the body needs an optimum amount of oxygen and nutrients to function effectively. Notice what the different muscle groups feel like when they are tensed, and where the tension radiates, if at all, and note the difference when you release the tension. Hold the muscle contraction a few seconds. Do each exercise once, repeating it only if necessary to become fully aware of the tension and release.

1. Flex your feet (bend them up toward you) at the ankle joints; release.
2. Flex feet again, and also straighten legs and tense thigh muscles; release.

3. Squeeze buttocks together; release.
4. Pull in abdomen; release.
5. Clench hands into fists and straighten arms, tensing muscles; release.
6. Shrug shoulders up toward ears; release.
7. Press head back down into pillow; release.
8. Wrinkle up face, clench teeth, and push tongue against them; release.

BLENDING TOGETHER

Have the person who will later be helping you through labor stroke, touch, or massage the parts you have just learned to relax. Release any residual tension into the warmth and pressure of your partner's hands. It is important to say how you prefer to be stroked or massaged. Be specific about how much pressure to use and where you want it. Reverse roles so that each knows the other's.

CREATING A POSITIVE SELF-IMAGE

Pregnancy, like adolescence, is likely to be a time of mercurial highs and lows for you, when your feelings about yourself are greatly affected by the changes that are taking place in your body. Your self-image is not only vulnerable to negative misgivings; it is also particularly susceptible to affirmative conditioning. This offers you the opportunity to actively build the high self-esteem that will benefit you not only in childbirth, when it is so essential to a good experience, but throughout your life. You can use the power of thought—the most creative tool you have—to promote the positive. Compose several affirmative statements and write them down 20 to 30 times a day: for example, "I, Joan, am beautiful during this pregnancy"; "My birth experience will be a perfect one for me and my family"; "I, Susan, have a body that functions effectively." Eventually simply through repetition your affirmations will displace any doubts, fears, or old misconceptions you may have.

Posture and Body Mechanics

There are two important reasons to be especially aware of your posture and the way you use your body in your regular activities during your pregnancy:

1. The hormone relaxin is produced. True to its name, it relaxes the ligaments and soft tissues in the body, to enable the pelvis to open up gently and accommodate the birth more readily. As the hormone is not selective but affects all parts of the body, it is important to take special care not to strain your back or overstretch any ligaments or joints.

2. As pregnancy progresses, the increased body weight shifts your center of gravity forward, making postural readjustment essential, especially to protect the back. The expanding uterus stretches and weakens the abdominal muscles as well as displacing the abdominal contents, pushing the diaphragm up and making breathing more difficult. It also pushes on major blood vessels, sometimes impeding circulation. Good body mechanics will help your body accommodate graciously to these changes and prevent muscle imbalance.

DAILY DO'S AND DON'TS

- Maintain a slight pelvic tilt by tightening your abdominal muscles and tucking the buttocks under. Keep your knees relaxed and and your feet at right angles to the lower legs. Keep your shoulders back, with the top of your head reaching for the ceiling, and your chin level. Don't stand with stiff knees, swayed back, or chin thrust forward.
- Keep everyday work at elbow level rather than reaching up above shoulders. Step up on a stool to avoid unnecessary reaching. Don't sway your back by reaching too high.

- To avoid backstrain place one foot on a stool when working in a standing position. Don't stand swaybacked, resting on ligaments.
- When you must lift an object bend at hips and knees, keeping your back straight as you rise by tucking your bottom in and straightening your knees and hips. Don't bend at the waist.
- Sit on a chair low enough to have your knees higher than your hips to prevent sway back. Sit up from a lying-down position by bending your knees up and rolling to your side, using your hands to push yourself up.
- Use a bedboard if your mattress is not a firm one.

Exercises During Pregnancy

Most authorities agree that with a normal pregnancy, any physical activity you were used to before pregnancy can be continued as long as you do not become fatigued, do not feel any stress or strain, and are in no obvious danger of falling, slipping, or otherwise hurting yourself. The exercises below are specifically created to condition your body for the hard work of labor and delivery and help it return to its pre-pregnancy state more rapidly. They should be practiced conscientiously from the beginning of pregnancy. But first consult your physician or midwife to be sure they are appropriate for you.

You will need a firm surface, such as a carpeted floor. Try to exercise as smoothly and rhythmically as possible. There should never be any discomfort or straining. You should always stop before reaching the point of fatigue. Unless otherwise indicated, start with 5 repetitions; gradually add one every other day until you are doing 10 to 15 a day. In order not to overtire any group of muscles, alternate exercises from each group. Do 20 to 30 minutes of exercise per day, in two or three sessions of 10 to 15 minutes each.

Pelvic Floor (Kegel) Exercises

The pelvis is the bony basin housing the important pelvic organs. The pelvic floor, or perineum, is slung like a hammock, forming the bottom of this basin, and is therefore a very important group of muscles. Besides supporting the pelvic organs, it controls the openings of the vagina, urethra, and rectum. Throughout life the perineum is subjected to various stresses and strains. These can be as simple as increased abdominal pressure when laughing, coughing, or sneezing; greater pressure when straining during a stool; greater still with the excess weight of the uterus during pregnancy and the stretching during delivery. A lax pelvic floor can lead to a condition known as stress incontinence, a leakage of urine with stress. A toned, supple pelvic floor which you are able to contract and release voluntarily enables you to give birth more easily. (It also will enhance sexual pleasure for both partners during pregnancy or at any other time.)

The muscles of the pelvic floor form a figure 8, with the urethra and vagina occupying one loop of the 8 and the anus the other. Cross your legs and squeeze them together, tightening your buttocks. Simultaneously pull up and tighten the muscles between your legs as though you need to urinate but have to wait. Once you are sure you can feel the muscles around the vagina and anus contract, it is important to confine the contraction to these muscles, releasing muscle tension everywhere else. Since it is easier to contract the muscles around the anus, concentrate on tightening the muscles all the way up the vagina.

Once in a while, try stopping and starting the flow of urine on a partially empty bladder. You can also try imagining the pelvic floor as an elevator. Go up four floors, contracting one floor at a time and not letting go in between floors. Then descend floor by floor, going all the way down to the basement. At this point the perineum will bulge downward and the vaginal lips part slightly if you purse your mouth and blow out as if blowing up a balloon that is difficult to blow up. (This puts the pelvic floor in a good position during pushing or internal examinations.) Finally return to the first floor, the correct posture for these muscles during everyday activities. Do at least 5 of these contractions 10 times a day.

Practice the pelvic floor exercises first when you are lying down; soon you will be able to do them sitting, then standing.

Circulatory Exercises

Goal: To improve circulation in the legs and help or prevent swollen ankles and varicose veins.

Position: Lying on back, head on pillow, legs elevated and supported 45 degrees by an inverted chair or loosely bent with a pillow under the knees.

Foot Pumping: Flex feet (toward you) and extend (back), moving only at the ankles. Repeat 30 times.

Ankle Circling: Separate legs slightly. Rotate both feet at once in circles as large as possible. Move them only at the ankles, without raising your legs off their support. Rotate clockwise 15 times; counterclockwise 15 times.

Thigh and Buttock Press: Press thighs together, straighten knees, and contract buttock muscles, as though pressing a thin paper between them. Hold 5 seconds and release.

Abdominal Exercises

Goal: To strengthen and tone the abdominal muscles.

Position: Lying on back, knees bent, feet flat on floor.

Pelvic Tilt (Rocking the Baby): Place one hand under the hollow of your back. Place the other hand on the rim of the hip bone. Slowly tightening abdominal and buttock muscles, flatten your hand against the floor by pushing it down with the small of your back. You will feel your hip bones rock back as you "rock your baby" into its pelvic cradle. Breathe out as you contract the abdominal muscles; maintain the contraction a few seconds; then relax gently and breathe in. Be sure not to arch the back upward.

Progression: Do the same exercise with your legs straight; then while kneeling on all fours (helps back discomfort); then in standing position.

Curl-up: Do pelvic tilt and breathe out. Stretch hands out in front of you, reaching for your knees. Slowly curl up, tucking your chin in first, and come up, vertebra by vertebra, lifting your head and shoulders off the ground as far as you comfortably can but not more than 45 degrees. If the abdominal muscles bulge in the middle when you rise, press against them with your hands, raising only your head, and work at pulling in your abdomen to control the bulge. It is very important to do this exercise slowly. Never jerk up suddenly.

Candle Blowing: Blow out, as though extinguishing a candle 12 inches in front of you, and tighten abdominal muscles firmly. Hold a few seconds, then release gently.

Pelvic Swinging: Gently lower both knees to one side with the bottom leg touching the floor, or as low as is comfortable. Raise them back to the vertical position and repeat on the other side.

Hip Hiking: Straighten one leg, keeping the other knee bent. Shorten it from the hip by hitching it up toward your waist, keeping the knee straight and the foot flexed at right angles to the leg. Reverse the procedure, stretching the leg out again. Repeat 10 times with each leg.

Progression: Do the same exercise while kneeling; then in standing position (duck walk).

Inner Thigh Stretching

Goal: To make the position of delivery more comfortable.

Position: Sitting with the knees bent, soles of the feet together and held close to crotch with one hand.

Knee Press: Push up with free hand under knee on same side, simultaneously using leg muscles to press knee down to floor. This makes the thigh and buttock muscles work hard while feeling the stretch of the inner thigh muscles. Hold a few seconds, release gently, and repeat on the other side.

Butterfly: Hold feet, soles touching, as close to your crotch as possible. Push knees downward, using only your leg muscles, and lean forward slightly until you feel the stretch on your inner thighs.

Breast Muscle Push

Goal: To strengthen the pectoral muscles.

Position: Sitting crosslegged on the floor.

Holding arms extended in front at right angles to shoulders, firmly grip each forearm with the opposite hand and push toward elbows as hard as you can, feeling the tightening of the pectoral muscles.

Neck and Shoulder Exercises

Goal: To help relaxation and prevent rounded shoulders.

Position: Sitting crosslegged on the floor.

Neck Rotation: Roll your head in a circle, first in one direction, then the other. It is important to take a lot of care with this exercise and do it very slowly.

Shoulder Rotation: Place hands on shoulders, right hand on right shoulder, left on left, and rotate elbows backward, making circles as large as possible.

Back Exercise

Goal: To strengthen spine and stabilize back.

Position: Kneeling on all fours, maintaining pelvic tilt.

Extend right arm and left leg in a straight line with your back. Repeat, using left arm and right leg. Do not lift arm and leg higher than the level of your back.

Foot Exercises

Goal: To strengthen the muscles of the feet and help prevent flattened arches, painful feet, and poor posture.

Position: Sitting in a chair; then standing.

Foot Arching: Push your toes down on the floor, keeping them straight, and try to raise the balls of your feet without curling your toes.

Toe Spreading: Spread your toes as far apart as you can; then relax.

Progression: Repeat both exercises in standing position.

Leg Exercise

Goal: To strengthen legs for more efficient lifting.

Climbing stairs or stepping on and off a stable platform, up to a foot high, will help accomplish this.

Phase II

The Lamaze method of childbirth preparation is not "natural childbirth." It is a psychological conditioning, combined with education and physical preparation for the birth event. It is also not childbirth without pain, although some women using the method experience very little or none. There can be a substantial amount, even when psychoprophylaxis, as the Lamaze method is often called, is conscientiously used. However, the important thing to remember is that the pain is never more than you will be able to deal with.

The Lamaze method cannot be thought of in terms of success or failure. Neither you nor it has failed should you require some form of medication or obstetrical intervention. But trusting in your ability to achieve a degree of comfort using the method will reduce the need for any such intervention or, if it becomes necessary, hold it to a minimum.

The exercises that follow should be started 8 to 12 weeks before the baby is due. They evolve from all here that has preceded them and become tools for you to adapt to your own childbirth needs. No two people, for example, breathe the same way during labor or give birth identically. Like you yourself, your experience will be unique.

Breathing

There are three types of breathing that can be adapted to any labor contraction. Think of them as gears, like first gear, second, and third in a stick-shift car. You move into a higher gear as a contraction gets stronger, and drop down to a lower, slower gear as it decreases in intensity. In first, the lowest gear, breathing is the deepest and slowest. It becomes shallower (higher in the chest) and faster as you move toward third. Consciously managing the rate and depth of your breathing has an added benefit: in focusing your concentration, it reduces pain.

Always try to keep your breathing rhythmical, exhaling after each breath no matter how shallow or fast. The rates of breathing you practice before childbirth are slower than those you may actually use during labor, when your uterus is contracting and you are utilizing large amounts of oxygen.

FIRST GEAR (*Low down in chest, just above waist*)

Speed: 6 to 9 breaths per minute.
Technique: Place hands just above waistline, feeling your ribs expand, as you inhale through your nose, and then retract, as you release and sigh out through slightly pursed lips. In timing this slow chest breathing, exclude the greeting breath, which will be

done at the beginning of a contraction, and the completion breath, done at the end of the contraction.

SECOND GEAR *(Middle of chest)*

Speed: Faster and shallower than slow chest, about 30 breaths per minute.

Technique: Inhale and exhale through mouth only, nose only, or both mouth and nose simultaneously—not as in first gear when you inhaled through your nose and exhaled through your mouth. Place hands on ribs at side of breasts. Part lips with a slight smile, placing tongue behind the top teeth if you prefer to breathe through your mouth. Your ribs will expand and lift slightly as you breathe in and recede as you breathe out.

THIRD GEAR *(Up in throat)*

Speed: Up to 60 breaths per minute—fastest and shallowest.

Technique: Inhale and exhale as in second gear. Part lips and smile slightly as in second gear. Place hands on neck, resting on collarbone. As you breathe, you will feel your collarbone gently rise and fall. It is sometimes helpful to make a small *hiss, hee,* or *tuh* sound as you exhale, and to emphasize the fourth exhale slightly to maintain an even rhythm.

NOTE: If you feel a little dizzy or tingly around your mouth or fingers or toes, you may have been breathing too deeply or too fast. This is called hyperventilation. Relax, slow down your breathing, and breathe into a small paper bag or your tightly cupped hands to increase the carbon dioxide level of your blood.

Focusing

As you breathe rhythmically, keep your eyes fixed on some one thing—a point in the room, or the eyes of your partner, who can help you focus and at the same time give you warm supporting messages.

Effleurage

This is a light abdominal massage, using the fingertips. It can be done by either you or your partner. When you do it during labor, the concentration required to keep hands and breathing in synchronization aids in reducing uterine sensations, and the stimulation of these superficial nerve endings helps to block the deeper discomfort. Maintain a steady rhythm, keeping it slow and relaxed even when doing the faster breathing. Effleurage is best done on the bare skin, using a little cornstarch to avoid irritation.

Start with the fingertips of both hands over the pelvic bone and draw them up lightly along both groins to the hip bones, back to the middle under the rib cage, and down to the starting point.

Effleurage can be done with one hand in a clockwise or counterclockwise direction. It can be done very low down, just above the pubic bone, in the groins, or on the thighs. (In labor a fetal monitor may prevent full abdominal massage.)

Selective Relaxation

Although these exercises are not done during labor, mastering them ahead of time will make it far easier for you to release tension in your body while the uterine muscle is contracting. If possible, practice with your labor partner, who should always use the same words to give you directions, so you become conditioned to both words and voice.

Settle into a comfortable nesting position. Your partner should check your relaxation. A relaxed person breathes slowly and rhythmically, with eyes focused and facial muscles relaxed. Each part of the body should feel heavy, each joint movable with no resistance.

Your partner gives a direction: for example, "Contract right arm." You then make a fist, lift the arm a little off its support, and tighten all its muscles. Concentrate on releasing any tension in the rest of your body. After looking and feeling to make sure you are relaxed everywhere else, your partner instructs you to relax the arm and checks the result. Continue with the same exercise for your left arm, then your right leg, then your left leg.

Next you will contract two limbs while releasing the rest of your body. Your partner directs: "Contract left leg and left arm." After being checked and allowed to release, reverse to right arm and right leg; then contract both legs while releasing arms; finally, contract both arms while relaxing both legs. It is harder to contract opposites. Try contracting right arm and left leg while consciously releasing left arm and right leg; then switch to contracting left arm and right leg. Your partner should remember to check tension in neck, jaw, and face.

The Lamaze "Goody Bag"

Sometime during the final weeks of your preparation you should begin to collect the things that will be of aid and comfort to you and your partner during labor and delivery.

1. To freshen up with: Brush, comb, and cologne.
2. To warm you up or cool you down: Warm socks and a fan.
3. To focus on: A favorite picture or object.
4. To aid resting and comfort: Face cloth and extra pillows.
5. To moisten dry lips and mouth: Lip ice, breath freshener, ice chips, lollipops, a natural sea sponge (to suck when dipped in ice water), a lemon slice.
6. To nourish your partner: Food.
7. For hyperventilation: A very small paper bag.
8. For back labor: Tennis balls, ice pack, warm-water bottle.

Now you are ready to complete your own and your partner's training by rehearsing specific responses to your anticipated labor contractions, repeating the experience many times. Work on at least one of each kind of contraction in different positions every day. Your partner can help condition your responses by giving consistently expressed cues to signify a contraction's beginning and end, by monitoring your relaxation and breathing attentively, and by acting out the emotional and physical support that will be an important part of this wonderful collaboration.

The pages that follow are to give you a fuller understanding of the actual process and to provide a scenario for final preparation. Included also is a quick-reference chart summarizing Stage 1 of labor.

The Three Stages of Labor

Stage 1: *Effacement and Dilation*

The first stage of labor is concerned with the slow thinning out (effacement) and opening of the cervix till it is big enough for the baby's head to pass through. During labor your doctor may measure the progress of cervix dilation with the fingers, five fingers' width (10 centimeters or about 4 inches) being full dilation.

It is impossible to predict how long this stage will last. With first babies, it averages 8 to 12 hours; usually less with subsequent births, 4 to 9 hours. Your uterus, however, will not listen to statistics, and labor can sometimes take as little as ½ hour or last longer than 12 hours. It is worth remembering that labor is a series of contractions with intervals between, so even though yours may last 12 hours, you are probably really working only about 3½.

The first stage of labor can be divided into three parts: *early labor* (effacement and early dilation, o to 3 cm), *accelerated labor* (3 to 7 cm dilation), and *transition* (full dilation, 7 to 10 cm).

The second stage of labor is the birth of the baby, while the third stage is delivery of the placenta, or afterbirth.

EARLY LABOR

There are three signs to indicate you are in labor, and they can appear in any order.

Show: The first sign is often the expulsion of the plug of mucus from the neck of the cervix. You may notice some mucous discharge which will be streaked with a little red blood (if it happened a few hours before, it will have changed to a brownish color). If it happens around the time your baby is due to be born, contractions could start in a few hours to a few days.

Rupturing of the amniotic sac: Also called the breaking of the bag of waters, this can be the first thing that happens in labor, but usually it happens at the end of first stage, and sometimes only in the second stage. Your doctor or midwife may want to rupture the amniotic sac during labor to help speed up the contractions.

Contractions: These involuntary movements of the uterus shorten the uterine muscle fibers, pulling on the cervix to thin it out and dilate it. The sensations of the contractions are usually described as a tightening or menstrual cramp that seems to start low down on the abdomen over the pubic area and spreads toward the back. Some women experience contractions in their groin or thighs. In early labor contractions are mild to moderate, about 5 to 20 minutes apart and lasting from between 30 to 60 seconds. Gradually they get closer together, longer, and stronger, until they are about 30 to 90 seconds apart and 60 to 90 seconds long toward the end of labor. The pushing contractions are more comfortable, generally not more than 60 seconds long with about 2 minutes in between each contraction. (Toward the end of your pregnancy you may be aware of "practice" contractions of the uterus, called Braxton Hicks contractions. These can be strong enough to start thinning out and dilating the cervix even before you go into labor.)

The baby rotates during labor, from facing your left or right hip to facing the back of your pelvis, with its head placed well forward so that the smallest part—the crown—pushes down on your cervix, encouraging it to dilate. About 25 percent of women experience labor contractions in their back as a low dull backache that comes and goes. Occasionally this is because the baby turns to face your pubic bone, instead of your back, and its head presses against the soft tissue and nerves of your back. Labor tends to be longer with the baby in that position, and often more uncomfortable. (It may be necessary for the doctor to use forceps to help rotate the baby's head before birth.) A firm massage over the lower back sometimes helps minimize the discomfort, or, if it is severe, a fist or two tennis balls pressed into the area can counter the pressure of the baby's head. An ice pack or warm-water bottle can have a soothing effect. And any position that gets the baby off your back is helpful—side lying, kneeling on all fours, leaning against a wall, or sitting and leaning forward.

Riding a labor contraction is very similar to riding a wave at sea. Until transition, a contraction usually begins slowly, increases in intensity until it reaches a crest, and then subsides. Using your breathing and relaxation you can keep on top of the waves of your contractions, maintaining control the way a surfer does who, ready for a wave, catches it at the beginning, rides it to a crest, and slowly follows it down.

False labor vs. real labor: You are generally not in labor if your contractions do not increase in intensity over a period of time, even though they may be coming at regular short intervals. A good indication that you are in real labor is that your contractions get stronger and last longer. Keep as calm as possible. Don't rush off to the hospital too soon.

ACCELERATED OR ACTIVE LABOR

Now the contractions get stronger and come closer together,

and you will start working harder to stay in control. The time between them is best spent resting and consciously relaxing. A sign that you are in active labor is that you feel a need to use a higher gear of breathing and greater relaxation to stay in control.

TRANSITION

This is an intense but very short phase, normally lasting less than ½ hour. It completes the thinning and opening of the cervix so that you can start pushing the baby out.

You may find it hard to communicate and become very anxious. You may get angry with your labor assistants, telling them to leave when what you really want to say is "I am afraid. Please help me. Whatever you do, don't leave now." You may feel nauseated, may even throw up. Other signs of transition are feeling that you won't be able to control the contractions if they get any stronger, experiencing back labor for the first time, getting hot flushes or chills. Shaking and trembling of an arm or leg or the entire body is fairly common. (It is best to succumb to this, even encourage it, as it will relieve tension.) Between contractions you may find it difficult to relax, or you may feel very sleepy and even fall asleep. Your partner must wake you before the next contraction, or not let you sleep at all, lest it take you unawares.

You may feel an urge to push (because of the pressure of the baby's head on the rectum during transition) before the cervix is fully dilated. Some physicians prefer you to blow out rhythmically and slowly to prevent pushing; others feel that gentle pushing shortens transition and makes it more comfortable.

These powerful transition contractions are the most difficult to control and require a great deal of determination on your part and encouragement and active coaching from your partner. Try to view them as a challenge, knowing that you're almost there.

GENERAL ADVICE

Labor rarely follows a textbook pattern. But your preparation, practice, and conditioning will enable you to be relaxed enough to control any pattern your labor may follow. Start the breathing gears only if you need to in order to stay relaxed. Stay with the easiest, slowest level of breathing as long as possible, remembering that each stage is progressively more difficult and tiring. It is, however, always more sensible to use a higher gear of breathing, even early in labor, than to tense up and become fatigued. Don't feel that you *must* save the higher gears for stronger labor. In some labors, contractions start strongly and do not increase very much in intensity toward the end.

During your contractions, visualize your cervix opening progressively as they become stronger. Imagine your baby rotating and moving down the birth canal.

THE PARTNER'S ROLE

Throughout labor, it is important to provide both emotional and physical support. Try to maintain a calm, relaxed atmosphere and give the mother lots of love, support, and encouragement. This can be through body language—the way you look at her and touch her—or it can be verbal—"I love you," "You're beautiful," "I'm proud of you." Be sensitive to what she needs, whether it is to arrange pillows for her nesting position, or to sponge or stroke or massage her body, or to give her things to relieve a dry mouth. It may help to hold her very close to you and keep in rhythm with her breathing, gently cueing her to slow it down or speed it up.

Specifically, constantly monitor her contractions and help her with relaxation. Remind her to empty her bladder and change position occasionally. Remind her to start each contraction with a greeting breath and to keep her eyes on a fixed point or focused on you. Help keep her breathing rhythmical or remind her to use a different tool if she becomes tense and cannot relax. Count off 15-second intervals during contractions to give her an idea of where she is in them. Remind her to end each contraction with a completion breath. Remind her to move her feet up and down at the end of a contraction to discourage cramps.

Stage 2: Birthing

Once fully dilated and given the go-ahead to start pushing, many women feel wonderful. The contractions at this point are more comfortable, shorter, and farther apart. They usually don't last longer than 60 seconds, and there is a 1-to-3-minute break in between. The contractions slowly increase to a crest, then gradually fall off.

You can push your baby out as you kneel or squat, taking advantage of gravity. Or you can lie on your back with your knees bent, legs spread apart, back supported at 45 degrees, and pelvis flat. Or you can birth your baby in what is known as the lateral Sims's position, lying on your side and lifting your top leg up.

PUSHING

The actual pushing out of your baby is probably the hardest work you will ever do, but the most exhilarating and rewarding. Women who are not afraid, but are relaxed and enthusiastic about their pushing, report that there is no pain with it—only lots of pressure. At the end of a contraction, you may feel the head slip up a little. As your baby's head moves down and under the pubic bone, you may feel a burning splitting sensation in the vaginal area a few contractions before the baby is born. (If you put your thumb and forefinger in your mouth and spread them apart horizontally, the feeling is very similar.)

As the baby's head is presenting, your birth assistants will tell you to stop pushing. This allows the vagina to accommodate slowly to the size of your baby's head. Sometimes it may be necessary to make a small painless incision in the perineum to prevent the tearing of the perineal tissue. This is called an episiotomy.

Here is how to push: (1) As you feel a contraction begin, get into position, take two relaxed greeting breaths, and tilt pelvis back. (2) Take a third deep breath in, let a little out, and hold the rest. (3) With face and jaw totally relaxed while holding breath, push down and out through a released pelvic floor. You are contracting your abdominal muscles and bulging them forward slightly. Push according to the feeling of the contraction. When you need to take another breath, exhale and repeat steps 2 and 3 once or twice more during a contraction.

There is another, gentler way to push which is said to minimize or prevent hemorrhoids, strain of abdominal muscles, or need for episiotomy: After your two greeting breaths, take a third deep breath in. Through pursed lips, force the air out really slowly, contracting your abdominal muscles and bulging them forward slightly. It is almost like blowing up a balloon that is very difficult to start. You may make a groaning sound or hold your breath a little during parts of the contraction. Take another breath when you need to, and repeat till the end of the contraction. Once more you are pushing according to the feeling of the contraction.

Once a little of your baby's head is showing, you may be taken to the delivery room, where your legs will be supported by stirrups. When instructed not to push, open your mouth and pant, silently saying *ha ha ha ha* (laughing the baby out). You may then be asked to push a little more; then stop again; and so on, until your baby is born. Be sure to keep your eyes open for this splendid moment. Your labor partner takes a more passive role now, supporting you and acting as liaison between you and the other labor assistants.

Stage 3: Afterbirth

All that remains now is to bring out the placenta, and hardly anything need be said about this stage. It usually requires only one more push—and by now you have become an expert.

Phase III

The exercises you learned to do prenatally will help get your body back into shape during the postpartum weeks. Do some deep breathing (inhaling deeply through your nose and then exhaling by blowing out all the air you can), foot pumping, ankle circling, and pelvic floor exercises, beginning them on the same day your baby is born. Once or twice a day, lie flat on your stomach to encourage your uterus back to its normal position. (Some pillows under your abdomen and chest will prevent compression of your breasts.) On the next day add the pelvic swinging, pelvic tilt, and candle-blowing exercises. Soon thereafter add the curl-up (carefully and slowly) and hip hiking. Wait until the lochia (bleeding from placental site) has stopped before beginning the back and leg strengthening exercises.

Correct posture and body mechanics—especially in lifting—are very important now.

If you can possibly manage it, join an exercise class when your baby is five or six weeks old and the lochia has stopped completely. It is a good idea to find one that is especially for new mothers. The support and sharing with friends who are also involved with new parenting can make the difference between being overwhelmed by your new role and enjoying it to the fullest.

STAGE 1 OF LABOR

	TYPICAL CONTRACTION	TECHNIQUES	VARIATIONS IN CONTRACTIONS/ RESPONDING TECHNIQUES	MOTHER'S CONDITION, PARTNER'S ROLE
EARLY LABOR *Dilation*: 0–2 fingers or 3 cm *Effacement*: early *Duration*: variable	*Intensity*: mild to moderate *Shape*: gentle wave, rising slowly to crest, then subsiding *Duration*: 30–45 seconds, occasionally longer *Intervals between*: 5–20 minutes	Start contraction with greeting breath. First-gear breathing, 6–9 breaths. End with completion breath. Stay in first gear as long as possible.	May start with higher intensity. Be prepared to begin with or switch to higher breathing gear.	*Mother*: very excited, slightly anxious. Usually high energy level. *Partner*: help keep things calm; avoid rushing to hospital too soon.
ACCELERATED OR ACTIVE LABOR *Dilation*: 2 fingers/3 cm–4 fingers/7 cm *Effacement*: continuing *Duration*: 5–10 hours first baby, 2–6 hours subsequent babies, also very variable	*Intensity*: moderate to strong *Shape*: wave reaches higher crest, has longer sweep *Duration*: ± 60 seconds *Intervals between*: 2–5 minutes	Start with greeting breath, end with completion breath. Vary breathing as needed, starting with first gear, moving to second, then third if needed, as contraction strengthens, dropping back to second then first when able.	May need to go straight into second gear, letting breathing become shallower and faster until in third gear. Vary speed of third gear or use transition breathing as necessary. Alternatively, may need only first-gear breathing, or invent your own pattern.	*Mother*: working very hard, feeling good about ability to control strong contractions. *Partner*: help her to relax between and during contractions. Give lots of love and encouragement. Sponge brow, give ice chips, etc. (You will usually go to birthing facility

TRANSITION			
Dilation: 4 fingers/7 cm–5 fingers/10 cm Effacement: complete Duration: 15–30 minutes, rarely longer than 1 hour	Intensity: very strong, peaking at times Shape: starts suddenly, has several crests, ends abruptly Duration: 60–90 seconds up to 2 minutes Intervals between: 30–90 seconds	Quick greeting breath, 4–6 third-gear breaths, + 1 breath followed by 1 short sharp blowing out as if of a candle. Repeat pattern, ending contraction with completion breath. Changing your rhythm of breathing can help you stay in control, i.e., 4 breaths + blow; 10–20 seconds later, 5 breaths + blow; then 2 (or 6) breaths + blow, etc. Combat urge to push by blowing out rhythmically as needed.	Mother: can feel overwhelmed by contractions and extremely anxious; may feel nauseated, hot and cold; may tremble or shake. Loses ability to communicate. Finds it difficult to relax between contractions, feels there is no break between. Feels sleepy or falls asleep between contractions. Partner: breathe and count with her, help her focus. Remind her birth is close.

Suggested Reading

Benson, Herbert, M.D. *The Relaxation Response*. New York: William Morrow and Company, 1975.

Bing, Elisabeth. *Six Practical Lessons for an Easier Childbirth*, rev. ed. New York: Bantam Books, 1977.

Boston Women's Health Book Collective. *Our Bodies, Ourselves*, 2nd ed. New York: Simon and Schuster, 1976.

Brewer, Gail Sforza, and Tom Brewer, M.D. *What Every Pregnant Mother Should Know: The Truth About Diet and Drugs in Pregnancy*. New York: Random House, 1977.

Chabon, Irwin. *Awake and Aware: Participating in Childbirth Through Psychoprophylaxis*. New York: Delacorte (Dell), 1969.

Donovan, Bonnie, and Ruth Allen. *The Cesarian Birth Experience: A Practical, Comprehensive, and Reassuring Guide for Parents and Professionals*. New York: Beacon Press, 1977.

Elkins, Valmay Howe. *The Rights of the Pregnant Parent*, rev. ed. Toronto, Canada: Waxwing Production. New York: Shocken Books, 1980.

Ewy, Donna, and Roger Ewy. *Preparation for Childbirth: A Lamaze Guide*. New York: New American Library (Signet Books), 1972.

Feldman, Sylvia. *Choices in Childbirth*. New York: Grosset & Dunlap, 1978.

Jacobson, Edmund. *How to Relax and Have Your Baby*. New York: McGraw-Hill, 1959.

Kitzinger, Sheila. *The Experience of Childbirth*, 4th ed. New York: Penguin Books (Pelican), 1978.

Lamaze, Fernand. *Painless Childbirth*. London: Burke, 1958; New York: Simon and Schuster (Pocket Books), 1977.

Montagu, Ashley. *Touching: The Human Significance of the Skin*. New York: Columbia University Press, 1971.

Noble, Elizabeth. *Essential Exercises for the Childbearing Year: A Guide to Health and Comfort Before and After Your Baby Is Born*. Boston: Houghton Mifflin Company, 1976.

Rakowitz, Elly, and Gloria S. Rubin. *Living with Your New Baby: A Postpartum Guide for Mothers and Fathers*. New York: Franklin Watts, 1978; Berkley, 1980.

Stewart, David, and Lee Stewart, eds. *Twenty-first Century Obstetrics Now*, vols. 1 and 2. (Transcription of the 1977 conference of the National Association of Parents and Professionals for Safe Alternatives in Childbirth.) Marble Hill, Mo.: NAPPSAC (P.O. Box 267, Marble Hill, Missouri 63764), 1978.

Techniques and Theories of the Psychoprophylactic Method of Childbirth. Washington, D.C.: American Society for Psychoprophylaxis in Obstetrics (Suite 200, 1411 K Street NW, Washington, D.C. 20005), 1980.

Wright, Erna. *The New Childbirth*. London: Tandem Books, 1964; New York: Simon and Schuster (Pocket Books), n.d.